T0073193

Praise for Who Shall Live? Health, Economics and Social Choice (3rd Edition)

"Vic Fuchs' *Who Shall Live?* is the most important book ever on health economics. It has inspired us all these many years, and it is terrific to see a new edition, post-Obamacare and post-pandemic."

Sir Angus S. Deaton
Recipient of the Nobel Prize in Economics 2015

"In considering the great health challenges of our time Victor Fuchs' work remains more important than ever. In the third edition, Fuchs' seminal text has been expanded to reflect recent policy and politics. It remains essential reading to better understand the complex interaction between social determinants, health and health care costs."

Victor J. Dzau, MD
President, National Academy of Medicine

"The problems addressed in this classic book, especially unequal access to health care, rising costs, and poor health outcomes, are just as relevant now as they were when the first edition appeared in 1974. The third edition includes updated analyses and materials about the most significant health policy questions."

Janet Currie
President-elect American Economic Association 2023

"Few, if any, social scientists have had more influence on thought and action in health care policy than Victor Fuchs. His greatest contribution may well be his prescient 1974 masterpiece, *Who Shall Live?*. Fuchs and Eggleston have updated this work and anyone who cares about health care policy should study this book, master its messages, and act."

Donald M. Berwick, MD
Former Administrator of the Centers for Medicare
and Medicaid Services (CMS)

"*Who Shall Live?* is the first book I read on health economics, and it is still the best. Few economists of any stripe are as wise as Fuchs and I thoroughly welcome this update of his classic text."

Anne C. Case
Professor of Economics and Public Affairs,
Emeritus, Princeton University

"Two decades since being assigned *Who Shall Live?* as foundational reading for my Ph.D. in Health Policy, I urge my students in the Medical School and the Graduate School of Business to read this compact up-to-date new edition to better prepare for reform of US health care."

Sara Singer
Professor of Medicine, Stanford University

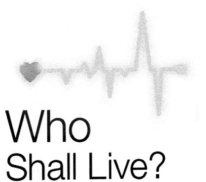

Who
Shall Live?

Health, Economics and Social Choice

3rd Edition

Selected other books by Victor Fuchs

Author

The Service Economy (1968)

How We Live (1986)

Women's Quest for Economic Equality (1988)

The Future of Health Policy (1993)

Health Economics and Policy (2018)

Editor

Production and Productivity in the Service Industries (1969)

Policy Issues and Research Opportunities in Industrial Organization (1972)

Essays in the Economics of Health and Medical Care (1972)

The Economics of Physician and Patient Behavior (with Joseph P. Newhouse, 1978)

Economic Aspects of Health (1982)

Individual and Social Responsibility: Child Care, Education, Medical Care, and Long-term Care in America (1996)

VICTOR R. FUCHS
KAREN EGGLESTON

Stanford University, USA

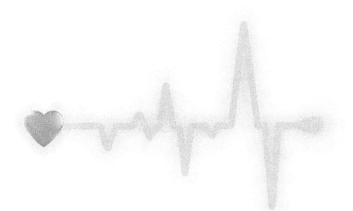

Who
Shall Live?

Health, Economics and Social Choice

3rd Edition

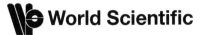

World Scientific

NEW JERSEY · LONDON · SINGAPORE · BEIJING · SHANGHAI · HONG KONG · TAIPEI · CHENNAI · TOKYO

Published by

World Scientific Publishing Co. Pte. Ltd.

5 Toh Tuck Link, Singapore 596224

USA office: 27 Warren Street, Suite 401-402, Hackensack, NJ 07601

UK office: 57 Shelton Street, Covent Garden, London WC2H 9HE

Library of Congress Cataloging-in-Publication Data

Names: Fuchs, Victor R, author. | Eggleston, Karen, author.
Title: Who shall live? : health, economics and social choice /
    Victor R Fuchs, Karen Eggleston, Stanford University, USA.
Description: 3rd Edition. | New Jersey : World Scientific, [2024] | Revised edition of
    Who shall live?, c2011. | Includes bibliographical references and index.
Identifiers: LCCN 2022053795 | ISBN 9789811268502 (hardcover) |
    ISBN 9789811269462 (paperback) | ISBN 9789811268519 (ebook) |
    ISBN 9789811268526 (ebook other)
Subjects: LCSH: Medical economics--United States. | Social medicine--United States. |
    Medical ethics--United States. | Medical policy--United States. | Health planning--United States. |
    Health care rationing--United States. | Health care reform--United States.
Classification: LCC RA410.53 .F82 2024 | DDC 338.4/73621--dc23/eng/20230120
LC record available at https://lccn.loc.gov/2022053795

British Library Cataloguing-in-Publication Data
A catalogue record for this book is available from the British Library.

For any available supplementary material, please visit
https://www.worldscientific.com/worldscibooks/10.1142/13204#t=suppl

Desk Editors: Soundararajan Raghuraman/Yulin Jiang

Typeset by Stallion Press
Email: enquiries@stallionpress.com

To my weekly Family Zoom
VF

To Adrian and Alanna, who shall live and thrive
KE

About the Book

Since the first edition of *Who Shall Live?* (1974), over 100,000 students, teachers, physicians, and general readers from more than a dozen fields have found this book to be a reader-friendly, authoritative introduction to economic concepts applied to health and medical care.

Health care is by far the largest industry in the United States. It is three times larger than education and five times as large as national defense. In 2001, Americans spent over $12,500 per person for hospitals, physicians, drugs and other health care services and goods. Other high-income democracies spend one third less, enjoy three more years of life expectancy, and have more equal access to medical care.

In this book, each of the chapters of the original edition is followed by supplementary readings on such subjects as: "Social Determinants of Health: Caveats and Nuances", "The Structure of Medical Education — It's Time for a Change", and "How to Save $1 Trillion Out of Health Care".

The ten years following publication of the 2nd expanded edition in 2011 were arguably more turbulent for US health and health care than any other ten-year period since World War II. They span the implementation of the Affordable Care Act, the deepening opioid epidemic, and the physical, psychological, and socio-economic traumas of the COVID-19 pandemic.

An important new contribution to this book is to describe and analyze the changes in five sections: "The Affordable Care Act and the Uninsured", "Health Care Expenditures", "Health Outcomes", "The COVID-19 Pandemic", and "Health and Politics". This part includes 24 tables and figures.

This book will be welcomed by students, professionals, and life-long learners to gain increased understanding of the relation between health, economics, and social choice.

About the Authors

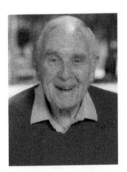

Victor R. Fuchs is the Henry J. Kaiser Jr., Professor of Economics and of Health Policy, Emeritus. He joined the Stanford faculty in 1974 in the Economics Department and the medical school. He has written extensively on the cost of medical care, on the determinants of health, and on health policy. Fuchs was president of the American Economic Association and is a member of the American Philosophical Society, the American Academy of Arts and Sciences, and the National Academy of Medicine. He was the first economist to receive the Distinguished Investigator Award from the Association for Health Services Research. The Victor R. Fuchs Award for lifetime contribution to health economics is awarded biennially by the American Society of Health Economists.

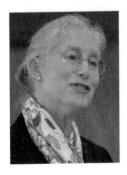

Karen Eggleston is a Senior Fellow at the Freeman Spogli Institute for International Studies at Stanford University, director of the Stanford Asia Health Policy Program at the Shorenstein Asia-Pacific Research Center, and a faculty research fellow of the economics of health program of the National Bureau of Economic Research. Previous books include *The Dragon, the Eagle, and the Private Sector* with John D. Donahue and Richard J. Zeckhauser, and *Welfare, Choice and Solidarity in Transition* with János Kornai.

Preface

The ten years following publication of the 2nd expanded edition of *Who Shall Live?* in 2011 were arguably more turbulent for U.S. health and health care than any other ten-year period since World War II. During 2012–2021, the first few years saw the implementation of the Affordable Care Act (ACA, or "Obamacare"). The last two years experienced the physical, psychological, and socio-economic traumas of the COVID-19 pandemic. Between the implementation of ACA and the pandemic, the opioid epidemic spread, and Donald Trump became President. Trump tried but failed to repeal the Affordable Care Act. Neither the opioid epidemic nor the COVID-19 pandemic has been curbed as this edition goes to press.

This edition of *Who Shall Live?* consists of three parts. The first is the original text of *Who Shall Live?* reprinted except masculine terms are replaced by gender-neutral language. The book's emphasis on problems of high cost, unequal access, and disappointing health outcomes is as relevant as this book goes to press as in 1974, as is the discussion of the strengths (and limitations) of economics in analyzing these problems.

The second part is a selection of our supplementary publications since 2011, which have been added to provide additional information and perspectives about health economics and health policy for the individual chapters of *Who Shall Live?*

The third part summarizes and discusses important data covering the health economy and health policy in the years 2012–2021. The discussions are grouped into five sections: The Affordable Care Act and the Uninsured, Health Care Expenditures, Health Outcomes, The COVID-19 Pandemic, and Health and Politics. The third part includes 24 tables and figures.

Contents

Part 1
Who Shall Live?

Health and Economics

> The Theory of Economics does not furnish a body of settled conclusions immediately applicable to policy. It is a method rather than a doctrine, an apparatus of the mind, a technique of thinking which helps its possessor to draw correct conclusions.
>
> JOHN MAYNARD KEYNES
> Introduction to the
> *Cambridge Economic Handbooks*

The problems are all around us: a parent searching frantically for someone to see a sick child; a crippling disease that puts a family hopelessly in debt; a tenfold increase in deaths from emphysema* since 1955; a doubling of Blue Cross rates in just a few years. The list could be extended almost without limit.

If the problems are numerous and varied, so are the proposed solutions. National health insurance, health maintenance organizations, public utility regulation of hospitals, expansion of medical schools, stricter control of drugs — these are some of the panaceas that have been offered to meet the "crisis" in health care.

Amid the emotion-laden debates that have surrounded these topics, it is not easy for the concerned layperson, government official, businessperson, student, labor leader, or even health professional to define the problems, acquire the necessary facts, and understand the critical individual and social choices that must be made.

To assist in this process is the primary purpose of this book. In it I try to distill analyses and conclusions based on my research in health services over the past decade, my experience on a medical school faculty, first-hand observation of many innovative medical care organizations, and discussions with leading professionals in medicine, hospital administration, the drug industry, public health,

---

*Chronic obstructive disease of the lung.

and related fields. Most important, this book approaches the problems of health and medical care from a specific point of view — that of the economist.

The economic point of view is rooted in three fundamental observations about the world. The first is that resources are scarce in relation to human wants. It is hardly news that we cannot all have everything that we would like to have, but it is worth emphasizing that this basic human condition is not to be attributed to "the system," or to some conspiracy, but to the parsimony of nature in providing humankind with the resources needed to satisfy human wants. That inefficiency and waste exist in the economy cannot be denied. That some resources are underutilized is clear every time the unemployment figures are announced. That the resources devoted to war could be used to satisfy other wants is self-evident. The fundamental fact remains, however, that even if all these imperfections were eliminated, total output would still fall far short of the amount people would like to have. Resources would still be scarce in the sense that choices would still have to be made. Not only is this true now, but it will continue to be true in the foreseeable future. Some advances in technology (e.g., automated laboratories) make it possible to carry out current activities with fewer resources, but others open up new demands (e.g., for renal dialysis* or organ transplants) that put further strains on resources. Moreover, our *time,* the ultimate scarce resource, becomes more valuable the more productive we become.

The second observation is that resources have alternative uses. Society's human, natural, and technological resources can, in most instances, be used to satisfy many different kinds of wants. If we want more physicians, we must be prepared to accept fewer scientists, or teachers, or judges. If we want more hospitals, we can get them only at the expense of more housing, or factories, or something else that could use the same land, capital, and labor.

Finally, economists note that people do indeed have different wants, and that there is significant variation in the relative importance that people attach to them. The oft-heard statement, "Health is the most important goal," does not accurately describe human behavior. Everyday in manifold ways (such as overeating or smoking) we make choices that affect our health, and it is clear that we frequently place a higher value on satisfying other wants.

Given these three conditions, the basic economic problem is how to allocate scarce resources so as to best satisfy human wants. This point of view may be contrasted with two others that are frequently encountered. They are the *romantic* and the *monotechnic.* The romantic point of view fails to recognize the scarcity of resources relative to wants. The fact that we are constantly being confronted with the need to choose is attributed to capitalism, communism, advertising, the unions, war, unemployment, or any other convenient scapegoat.

---

*A machine process that cleans the patient's blood of the waste chemicals that the non-functioning kidneys are unable to remove.

Because *some* of the barriers to greater output and want satisfaction are clearly human-made, the romantic is misled into confusing the real world with the Garden of Eden. Because it denies the *inevitability* of choice, the romantic point of view is impotent to deal with the basic economic problems that face every society. Occasionally, the romantic point of view is reinforced by authoritarian distinctions regarding what people "need" or "should have." Confronted with an obvious imbalance between people's desires and the available resources, the romantic-authoritarian response may be to categorize some desires as "unnecessary" or "inappropriate," thus protecting the illusion that no scarcity exists.

The monotechnic point of view, frequently found among physicians, engineers, and others trained in the application of a particular technology, is quite different. Its principal limitation is that it fails to recognize the multiplicity of human wants and the diversity of individual preferences. Every problem involving the use of scarce resources has its technological aspects, and the contribution of those skilled in that technology is essential to finding solutions. The solution that is optimal to the engineer or physician, however, may frequently not be optimal for society as a whole because it requires resources that society would rather use for other purposes. The desire of the engineer to build the best bridge or of the physician to practice in the best-equipped hospital is understandable. But to the extent that the monotechnic person fails to recognize the claims of competing wants or the divergence of one's own priorities from those of other people, the advice from such a person is likely to be a poor guide to social policy.

The basic plan of this book is straightforward. Thus, the first chapter presents from an economic point of view the nation's major health care problems: high and rapidly rising costs, inequality and difficulties of access, and large disparities in health levels within the United States and between the United States and other countries. The discussion of these problems, and the subsequent analysis of the choices we must make, set the stage for a few central themes that run throughout the book.

The first theme is that the connection between health and medical care is not nearly as direct or immediate as most discussions would have us believe. True, advances in medical science, particularly the development of antiinfectious drugs in the 1930s, '40s, and '50s, did much to reduce morbidity and mortality. Today, however, differences in health levels between the United States and other developed countries or among populations in the United States are not primarily related to differences in the quantity or quality of medical care. Rather, they are attributable to genetic and environmental factors and to personal behavior. Furthermore, except for the very poor, health in developed countries no longer correlates with per capita income. Indeed, higher income often seems to do as much harm as good to health, so that differences in diet, smoking, exercise, automobile driving and other manifestations of "life-style" have emerged as the major determinants of health. Chapter 2 develops this theme in some detail.

Although it is the patient rather than the physician who has the major influence on health, the opposite is true regarding the cost of medical care. As we shall see in Chapter 3, it is the physician who, as "captain of the team," makes the key decisions (regarding hospitalization, surgery, prescriptions, tests, and X rays) that account for the bulk of medical care costs. Many of these decisions are not rigidly determined by "medical necessity," and, depending upon how medical care is paid for, utilization and costs can vary greatly. This theme is further elaborated in the chapters on hospitals (4), drugs (5), and medical care finance (6).

The relative unimportance of the physician in health and the great importance with respect to cost lead us naturally to a third theme — the folly of trying to meet the problem of access by training more M.D. specialists and subspecialists. The access problem involves mostly primary care* and emergency care — and could frequently be met with physicians' assistants, nurse clinicians, and other kinds of health professionals. The "doctor shortage" is far from universal, and in some specialties, such as surgery, there is actually a surplus. Furthermore, such surpluses, rather than reducing costs, actually raise them (see Chapter 3).

A fourth theme, concerning the payment for medical care (Chapter 6), is that there is no magic formula which can transfer the cost from individuals to government or business. If the American people want more medical care, they are going to have to pay for it through fees, insurance premiums, taxes, or, if the taxes are levied on business, higher prices. The choice of payment mechanism is not irrelevant, however, because of its implications for the poor, and its implications for the total cost of care.

The most central theme of the book is the necessity of choice at both the individual and social levels. We cannot have all the health or all the medical care that we would like to have. "Highest quality care for all" is "pie in the sky." We have to choose. Furthermore, while economics can help us to make choices more rationally and to use resources more efficiently, it cannot provide the ethics and the value judgments that must guide our decisions. In particular, economics cannot tell us how much equality or inequality we should have in our society (Chapters 1, 6, and the Conclusion).

A few words about what this book is *not* are also in order. Although I am a specialist in health economics, this book is not written for my fellow specialists. I have not attempted to fill in all the details or to argue exhaustively in support of every conclusion. I have tried very hard to get the main points right; indeed, to help the reader realize what the main points are. In a world that is becoming increasingly specialized, it is important to try to take a look at the "big picture," to reach an audience which, if not large, is certainly influential.

---

*The care given by practitioners who agree to serve as the first point of contact for the patients who need or think they need health services. It typically deals with the more common and relatively uncomplicated types of health problems.

This is not an "angry" book; neither is it a defense of the status quo. Surely there is much in the American health care scene to criticize, much that ought to be changed. But if the change is to be for the better, it should be based on an understanding of why things are the way they are. Anger often gets in the way of understanding. As Gordon McLachlan, a leading British health care expert, has written, "One of the major policy requirements for most Western societies today is to eschew the drama for awhile, and examine critically with scientific techniques the dogmas and cliches with which the policy-making for medical care has been encumbered."[1]

This book is not a directory of villains. It is simply not true that you can always recognize the "bad guys" by their white coats. Most health care problems are complex, and, except for my desire to avoid being too technical, the complexities are not evaded. Few simple solutions are presented, because, in my view, few exist. Some health care problems defy "solution." At most one can hope for understanding, adjustment, amelioration.

Although I have tried to avoid polemics, I have not tried to conceal my opinions or to present a balanced point of view on every issue. Other observers — indeed, other economists — may well reach conclusions different from mine. Some of the data are certainly open to alternative interpretations. More important, value judgments undoubtedly differ. My greatest hope is not that readers will uncritically accept all my conclusions, but that this book will help them reach their own with a firmer command of the facts and a clearer understanding of the relationships among health, economics, and social choice.

CHAPTER 1

Problems and Choices

> A rational man acting in the real world may be
> defined as one who decides where he will strike
> a balance between what he desires and what
> can be done. It is only in imaginary worlds that
> we can do whatever we wish.
>
> WALTER LIPPMANN
> *The Public Philosophy*

The Problems We Face

In recent years, almost every American family has become acutely aware of the soaring costs of medical care, the difficulties of access to physicians, and the mounting health problems of our society. According to many observers, the U.S. health care system is in "crisis." But a crisis is a turning point, a decisive or crucial point in time. In medicine the crisis is that point in the course of the disease at which the patient is on the verge of either recovering or dying. No such decisive resolution is evident with respect to the problems of health and medical care. Our "sick medical system," to use the headline of numerous magazine and newspaper editorials, is neither about to recover nor to pass away. Instead, the basic problems persist and are likely to persist for some time to come.

What are these problems? Many of them are related to the *cost* of care. Indeed, one close observer of the Washington scene has argued that "the medical 'crisis' ... is purely and simply a crisis of cost. The inflationary rise in medical costs is the key concern of congressmen and consumers, a fundamental political and economic fact of life for both."[1] Another category of problems concerns *access* to care; while a third major set involves the determinants of *health levels*. Let us look briefly at each of the problems in turn.

COST

In 1973 Americans spent an average of $450 per person for health care and related activities such as medical education and research. This was almost 8 percent of the GNP (the gross national product is the total value of all goods and services produced in the nation). Twenty years before, health care represented only 4.5 percent of the nation's output, and even as recently as 1962 the proportion was only 5.6 percent. Thus from 1963 to 1973 health expenditures rose at the rate of 10 percent annually while the rest of the economy (as reflected in the GNP) was growing at only 6 to 7 percent.

One often reads or hears that costs have become so high that the average family can no longer pay for health care and that some other way must be found to finance it. This is pure nonsense. The average family will always have to pay its share of the cost one way or the other. Payment may take many forms: fee-for-service, insurance premiums, or taxes. If the system is financed by taxes on business, then people pay indirectly, either through higher prices for the goods and services business produces or through lower wages. True, a highly progressive tax could result in some redistribution of the burden. But given the likely pattern of tax incidence, the only meaningful way to ease the cost burden on the average family is to moderate the increase in total expenditures.

Not only is *average* cost of health care high and growing at a rapid rate, but there is also the problem of *unusual* cost. It is clear that in any particular year a relatively small number of families make extensive use of health services, and if payment is on a fee-for-service basis, the cost to them is exceedingly high. Renal dialysis for one individual, for instance, may cost ten thousand dollars a year; some surgical procedures cost even more. But the remedy for this problem has been known for a long time — some form of insurance or prepayment. This will not help the *average*-cost problem — indeed, it would aggravate it if insurance were to induce additional utilization — but it does take care of those individuals who require unusually large amounts of care.

Note that these two cost problems have little to do with one another. If average costs were half their present levels or rising at half their present rate, some families would still experience mammoth medical care bills in any given year. Similarly, even if every family had complete protection against unusual costs through major-risk insurance, the problem of slowing the escalation of rising average costs would remain. They are separate problems and require separate solutions.

Why has average cost grown so rapidly, and what can be done about it? One useful approach is to realize that cost, measured by total expenditures, is equal to the *quantity* of care utilized multiplied by the *price* per "unit" of care. Utilization, measured by number of visits, prescriptions, tests, days in hospital, and the like, depends upon the *health condition* of the population as well as its *propensity to use health services* for any particular health condition. This propensity depends in part on the patient, who, in most instances, must initiate the care process and consent to its continuance. But it also depends on the physician who, because of presumed superior knowledge, is empowered by law and custom with the authority to make decisions concerning utilization. It is the physician who sends the patient to the hospital and then home, who recommends surgery, who orders tests and X-rays, and who prescribes drugs.

So much for utilization. What about price? The price of a given "unit" of medical care depends on the relative *productivity* (i.e., output per unit of input) of the labor and capital used to produce it and on the *prices paid* for this labor and capital. Productivity depends on such factors as the appropriateness of the scale and type of organization in question, on the amount of excess capacity, on technological advance, and on the effectiveness of incentives and training. Thus productivity is directly affected if a hospital is either too large or too small to be efficient, or if the community has more hospital beds than it needs, or if there are less expensive ways of performing laboratory tests.

Physicians can have considerable influence on productivity because of their broad powers of decision making. For instance, the physicians decide how many and what kinds of auxiliary personnel work with them in their practice. And committees of physicians make many of the critical decisions that affect productivity in the hospitals they are affiliated with. The patient can also affect productivity through cooperation and general behavior. For instance, a patient who gives a physician a full and reliable medical history and who complies with the latter's instructions regarding drugs and diet can contribute substantially to the efficiency of the care received. Furthermore, although the prices paid for labor and capital used in health care are largely governed by forces at work in the economy at large, special circumstances within the health field, such as the unionization of hospital employees, can affect wages and thus costs.

Any explanation for the rise in the average cost of health care and any proposal for containing or lowering this cost can be analyzed within the accounting framework just described, for nothing affects cost that does not first affect the health of the population, the propensity of people to use health services, the productivity of the factors of production (labor and capital) used in medical care, or the prices paid for those factors. It should be stressed, however, that this is an *accounting* framework; it cannot provide a behavioral explanation of cost change. That can only come through an analysis of the actual behavior of patients, physicians, hospital administrators, government officials, and other decision makers.

It is not easy to say how much of the increase in cost in the past decade is due to the increased quantity of health care and how much to higher prices. Price should refer to some well-defined unit of service, but in fact the "content" of a physician's visit, or of a day in the hospital, keeps changing over time. The official price index for medical care, which is an average of changes in the price of a hospital day, a physician visit, and other elements of care and is published by the U.S. Bureau of Labor Statistics, shows an annual increase of 5 percent since 1962. This implies that there was also a 5 percent annual increase in *quantity* of these goods and services over the same period (for the sum of the two must equal the 10 percent annual increase in total medical expenditures cited at the beginning of this section). But because the official price index makes little allowance for changes in health care *quality* (i.e., the effects on health or the amenities associated with care) it may give a misleading picture of the true changes in *quantity*. To the extent that the quality of care has increased, the price index is overstated; if quality has decreased, it is understated.

Part of what we know to be an increase in quantity is due to the growth of population which has been about 1 percent annually since 1962. The balance must reflect either an increased propensity to use health services or adverse changes in the health condition of the population because of pollution, smoking, increased numbers of accidents, and the like.

The price of medical care has been growing more rapidly than the overall price index and at about the same rate as the price index for all services. This reflects higher prices for the inputs used in medical care, particularly the labor of physicians, nurses, and other personnel. It also reflects our inability to increase productivity in health care as rapidly as in the economy as a whole.

Most proposals for medical care reform seek to contain costs, but there are important differences in the strategies proposed for accomplishing this. These strategies, which will be discussed in more detail in subsequent chapters, are introduced briefly here.

The first strategy looks to *changes in supply* to drive down price and ultimately cost. According to this view, a substantial increase in the number of hospitals and physicians would force significant reductions in charges and fees, presumably either by stimulating increases in productivity or decreases in prices and wages.

A second strategy would reduce utilization by *improving the health* of the population. Advocates of this approach argue that more preventive medicine, health education, and environmental improvements could reduce the need for hospitals, physicians, and drugs.

A third approach would depend upon administrative *controls and planning* to contain costs. Such devices as hospital planning councils, utilization review committees, and drug formularies fall into this category, as do more direct interventions such as wage and price ceilings. Some controls are intended to reduce utilization, others to improve productivity, and still others to limit prices paid to the factors of production.

A fourth strategy attempts to induce *greater cost-consciousness* in consumers by modifying health insurance to include substantial deductibles (amounts the patient must pay before the insurance becomes effective) and coinsurance (partial payment by the patient after the insurance becomes effective). The goal here is to reduce the propensity to use health services for any given health condition, and also to increase the consumer's incentive to maintain health.

Finally, there are those who look to the *physician to control costs*; changing the method of compensation, according to this strategy, would give the physician a strong incentive to do so. For instance, it is argued that payment on a capitation* basis, rather than fee-for-service, would reduce the number of unnecessary operations.

In order to evaluate these diverse strategies, one needs a good understanding of the determinants of health and of the workings of the health care market. My own view is that decentralized administrative controls and modification of patient behavior both have something to contribute, but I would put greatest emphasis on the physician. My reasons for emphasizing the physician as the key to controlling costs are developed in subsequent chapters.

ACCESS

The problems of access to health care fall into two main categories, which may be labeled "special" and "general." The special problems of access are those faced by particular groups in society — the poor, the ghetto dwellers, and the rural population. The general problem of access is one that is felt even by individuals and families who have enough income or insurance to pay for care and are not disadvantaged by reason of location or race. For them the problem is simply to get the kind of care they need when they need it.

The problems the poor face in getting access to medical care are similar to those they face in obtaining other goods and services. To be poor is, by definition, to have less of the good things produced by society; if they did not have less they would not be poor. There are many people, however, who argue that medical care is special, that access to care is a "right" and should not be dependent upon income. Opposed to this is the view that if one wishes to help the poor, the best way to do so is to give them more purchasing power and let *them* decide how they want to spend it. According to this view, it makes little sense to use hard-to-raise tax money to lift the poor up to some arbitrarily high standard of medical care while they have grievous deficiencies in housing, schooling, and other aspects of a good life. A more systematic look at this question is presented later in this chapter.

Poverty explains part of the access problem for the rural population, but not all of it. Even in rural areas with substantial purchasing power, the physician-population ratio is typically much lower than in the cities. This is true not only in the United States but in almost every country in the world. It is true in Israel, which has a very large supply of physicians because of immigration; it is true in Sweden, which is frequently said to have a model health care system; it is even true in the Soviet Union, where physicians are government employees and supposedly must practice wherever they are sent.

The reason for the access problem in rural areas is very clear: physicians prefer to practice in highly urbanized areas. They do so partly for professional reasons such as the desire to practice with colleagues, use up-to-date facilities, and

*A system in which the physician receives a fixed amount per patient per year regardless of the amount of care actually delivered.

concentrate on a specialty. They also generally prefer the educational, cultural, and recreational facilities available for themselves and their families in metropolitan areas.

What, if anything, to do about the rural access problem is less clear. Should physicians be forced to go to rural areas? Should they be bribed to go there with very high incomes financed by taxes on citydwellers? One popular proposal is to subsidize medical education on condition that the student promises to practice in a rural area. In the absence of any demonstration that health is worse in rural areas, however, I do not see any strong case for adopting special measures aimed solely at changing physicians' location decisions. If, however, such decisions were to be influenced by broader programs aimed at rural poverty, or at a wider dispersion of the population, that would be a different matter.

The access problem for Blacks and some other minority groups is largely a question of poverty. Many members of minority groups with adequate incomes and insurance do not experience any unique problems with respect to health care. Where discrimination in housing is severe, however, and middle- and upper-income Blacks are locked into low-income ghettos, they probably will experience access problems because the supply of services is geared to the low average level of income in the area. The best solution for this problem is to eliminate discrimination in housing. Another distinct problem arises when Blacks (or Chicanos or Indians) prefer to be treated by other Blacks (or Chicanos or Indians); this can only be solved by increasing the number of health professionals from these minority groups.

The *general* problem of access, which will receive considerable attention in this book — especially in Chapter 3, where we discuss the physician — is a complex phenomenon that in the broadest sense represents a failure of the medical care market to match supply and demand. While the term *general problem* implies that it is experienced by the population generally and not only by particular groups, it must not be thought that the problem is general in the sense of applying to all kinds of physicians. As already mentioned in the Introduction (and as Chapter 3 will make clear), there are actually substantial surpluses of some types of physician specialists, such as surgeons. The general problem of access exists mainly with respect to primary care, emergency care, home care, and care outside customary working hours. And so the solution, as we shall see in Chapter 3, does not lie in simply increasing the number of physicians.

HEALTH LEVELS

Concern about health levels in the United States primarily takes two forms. First, there is concern that health levels in this country are not as high as in many other developed nations. The principal evidence for this is found in comparisons of age-specific death rates and of life expectancies (life expectancy is a summary measure of these death rates). The excess of death rates in the United States over those elsewhere is, in some cases, striking. For instance, the death rate for males ages 45 to 54 is almost double the Swedish rate. Of every hundred males in the United States who turn 45, only ninety will see their fifty-fifth birthday. In Sweden, ninety-five will survive the decade. Granted, there are many dimensions of health besides mortality, but the lack of adequate measures precludes their use for comparisons among populations. In any case, there seems little reason to believe that examination of these other dimensions would reverse conclusions based on mortality. Most deaths, after all, are preceded by illness, either physical or mental.

Infant mortality is another frequently used index of health. This indicator usually falls as income rises, but the United States, which has the highest per capita income in the world, does not have the lowest infant death rate. Indeed, the rate in this country is one-third higher than in the Scandinavian countries and the Netherlands.

The other principal cause for concern regarding health levels is that they vary greatly among different groups in the United States. For instance, the disparity between Whites and Blacks is very great. Black infant mortality in this country is almost double the White rate, and Black females ages 40–44 have two-and-one-half times the death rate of their White counterparts. Other minority groups (e.g., the Indians) also have very poor health levels, while still others, such as the Japanese and the Mormons, enjoy levels that are considerably above the national average.

The most important thing to realize about such differences in health levels is that they are usually *not* related in any important degree to differences in medical care. Over time the introduction of new medical technology has had a significant impact on health, but when we examine differences among populations at a given moment in time, other socioeconomic and cultural variables are now much more important than differences in the quantity or quality of medical care.

Medical advances beginning in the 1930s and extending through the late 1950s brought about significant improvements in health, especially through the control of infectious diseases. These advances have been widely diffused among and within all developed countries and even some of the less developed ones. For more than a decade, however, the impact of new medical discoveries on overall mortality has been slight; indeed, the death rate for U.S. males at most ages, except the very young and the very old, has actually been rising. The chief killers today are heart disease, cancer, and violent deaths from accidents, suicide, and homicide. The behavioral component in all these causes is very large, and until now medical care has not been very successful in altering behavior.

The preceding discussion of the problems of cost, access to medical care, and health levels indicates why there is so much concern about health care and so many proposals for changes in its organization and financing. In appraising such proposals it is useful to keep in mind the central economic problem of allocating scarce resources among competing needs. The promises of the planners and the panaceas of the politicians, then, must be seen against the reality of difficult choices.

The Choices We Must Make

An appreciation of the inevitability of choice is necessary before one can begin to make intelligent plans for health-care policy, but more than that is required. Some grasp of the variety of levels and kinds of choices we make is also essential. All of us, as individuals, are constantly confronted with choices that affect our health. In addition, some choices must be exercised collectively, through government.

HEALTH OR OTHER GOALS?

The most basic level of choice is between health and other goals. While social reformers tell us that "health is a right," the realization of that "right" is always less than complete because some of the resources that could be used for health are allocated to other purposes. This is true in all countries regardless of economic system, regardless of the way medical care is organized, and regardless of the level of affluence. It is true in the communist Soviet Union and in welfare-state Sweden, as well as in our own capitalist society. No country is as healthy as it could be; no country does as much for the sick as it is technically capable of doing.

The constraints imposed by resource limitations are manifest not only in the absence of amenities, delays in receipt of care, and minor inconveniences; they also result in loss of life. The grim fact is that no nation is wealthy enough to avoid all avoidable deaths. The truth of this proposition is seen most clearly in the case of accidental deaths. For instance, a few years ago an airplane crashed in West Virginia with great loss of life. Upon investigation it was found that the crash could have been avoided if the airport had been properly equipped with an electronic instrument-landing device. It was further found that the airport was fully aware of this deficiency and that a recommendation for installation of such equipment had been made several months before the crash — and turned down because it was decided that the cost was too high.

Traffic accidents take more than fifty thousand lives each year in the United States, and because so many of the victims are young or middle-aged adults,* the attendant economic loss is very high. As a first approximation, the relative economic cost of death can be estimated from the discounted future earnings of the deceased if the person had lived. According to such calculations, the death of a person at twenty

---

* The motor accident death rate reaches its peak in the late teens and early twenties.

or thirty is far more costly than death at seventy. Many of these traffic deaths could be prevented, but some of the most effective techniques, such as the elimination of left turns, are extremely expensive to implement. The same is true of deaths from other causes — many of them are preventable if we want to devote resources to that end. The yield may be small, as in the case of a hyperbaric chamber* that costs several million dollars and probably saves a few lives each year, but the possibilities for such costly interventions are growing. Current examples include renal dialysis, organ transplants, and open-heart surgery. Within limits set by genetic factors, climate, and other natural forces, every nation chooses its own death rate by its evaluation of health compared with other goals.

But surely health is more important than anything else! Is it? Those who take this position are fond of contrasting our unmet health needs with the money that is "wasted" on cosmetics, cigarettes, pet foods, and the like. "Surely," it is argued, "we can afford better health if we can afford colored telephones." But putting the question in this form is misleading. For one thing, there are other goals, such as justice, beauty, and knowledge, which also clearly remain unfulfilled because of resource limitations. In theory, our society is committed to providing a speedy and fair trial to all persons accused of crimes. "Justice delayed is justice denied." In practice, we know that our judicial system is rife with delays and with pretrial settlements that produce convictions of innocent people and let guilty ones escape with minor punishment. We also know that part of the answer to getting a fairer and more effective judicial system is to devote more resources to it.

What about beauty, natural or manmade? How often do we read that a beautiful stand of trees could be saved if a proposed road were rerouted or some other (expensive) change made? How frequently do we learn that a beautiful new building design has been rejected in favor of a conventional one because of the cost factor? Knowledge also suffers. Anyone who has ever had to meet a budget for an educational or research enterprise knows how resource limitations constrain the pursuit of knowledge.

What about more mundane creature comforts? We may give lip service to the idea that health comes first, but a casual inspection of our everyday behavior with respect to diet, drink, and exercise belies this claim. Most of us could be healthier than we are, but at some cost, either psychic or monetary. Not only is there competition for resources as conventionally measured (i.e., in terms of money), but we are also constantly confronted with choices involving the allocation of our time, energy, and attention. If we are honest with ourselves there can be little doubt that other goals often take precedence over health. If better health is our goal, we can achieve it, but only at some cost.

---

*A specially constructed facility for raising the oxygen content of air in order to treat more effectively certain rare diseases.

Stating the problem in this fashion helps to point up the difference between the economist's and the health professional's view of the "optimum" level of health. For the health professional, the "optimum" level is the highest level technically attainable, regardless of the cost of reaching it. The economist is preoccupied with the *social optimum,* however, which is defined as the point at which the value of an additional increment of health exactly equals the cost of the resources required to obtain that increment. For instance, the first few days of hospital stay after major surgery might be extremely valuable for preventing complications and assisting recovery, but at some point the value of each additional day decreases. As soon as the value of an additional day's stay falls below the cost of that day's care, according to the concept of social optimum, the patient should be discharged, even though a longer stay would be desirable if cost were of no concern. The cost reminds us, however, that those resources could be used to satisfy other goals.

The same method of balancing *marginal benefit* and *marginal cost** is equally applicable in choosing the optimum number of tests and X rays, or in planning the size of a public health program, or in making decisions about auto-safety equipment. Indeed, the concept of margin is one of the most fundamental tools in economics. It applies to the behavior of consumers, investors, business firms, or any other participant in economic life. Most decisions involve choosing between a little more or a little less — in other words, comparing the marginal benefit with the marginal cost. The optimum level is where these are equal and the marginal cost is increasing faster (or decreasing slower) than the marginal benefit.

MEDICAL CARE OR OTHER HEALTH PROGRAMS?

But weighing individual and collective preferences for health against each and every other goal is only the first choice. There is also a range of choices within the health field itself. Assume that we are prepared to devote x amount of resources to health. How much, then, should go for medical care and how much for other programs affecting health, such as pollution control, fluoridation of water, acci-dent prevention, and the like? There is no simple answer, partly because the ques-tion has rarely been explicitly asked. In principle, the solution is to be found by applying the economist's rule of "equality at the margin." This means relating the incremental yield of any particular program to the incremental cost of the program and then allocating resources so that the yield per dollar of additional input is the same in all programs.

Expenditures for any type of health-related activity, be it a hyperbaric chamber for a hospital or a rat-control program in the ghetto, presumably have some favor-able consequences for health which can be evaluated. It is not easy to measure these consequences, but we could do a lot better than we are doing and thus con-tribute to more rational decision making.

---

* Marginal (or incremental) benefits and costs are those resulting from small changes in inputs.

Hypothetical Illustration of Distinction between Average
and Marginal Benefit

	EXPENDITURES	VALUE OF BENEFITS	AVERAGE BENEFIT PER DOLLAR OF EXPENDITURES	MARGINAL BENEFIT PER DOLLAR OF EXPENDITURES
Cancer Screening Program	$10,000	$50,000	$5.00	$3.00
	20,000	80,000	4.00	2.00
	30,000	100,000	3.33	2.00
	40,000	120,000	3.00	1.00
	50,000	130,000	2.60	.50
	60,000	135,000	2.25	
Antismoking Program	$10,000	$30,000	$3.00	$2.00
	20,000	50,000	2.50	2.00
	30,000	70,000	2.33	2.00
	40,000	90,000	2.25	1.50
	50,000	105,000	2.10	1.00
	60,000	115,000	1.92	

Note that decisions about expanding or contracting particular programs should be based on their respective *marginal* benefits, not their *average* benefits. Thus, while a particular health program — say, screening women once a year for cervical cancer — may be particularly productive (that is, yield a high average benefit per dollar of cost), it does not necessarily follow that expanding that program twofold — for example, screening women twice a year — will be twice as productive. Some other program — say, an antismoking advertising campaign — might not show as high an average return as the screening program, yet the marginal return to *additional* expenditures might exceed that obtainable from additional cancer screening. In the following hypothetical numerical example, cancer screening has a higher average benefit than the antismoking campaign at every expenditure level, but the *incremental* yield from additional expenditures at any level above $40,000 is higher for the antismoking program. Thus if both programs were at the $40,000 level, it would be preferable to expand the second one rather than the first.

An objection frequently raised to such an approach is that "we can't put a price on a human life." One answer to this is that we implicitly put a price on lives whenever we (or our representatives) make decisions about the coverage of a health insurance policy, the installation of a traffic light, the extension of a food stamp program, or innumerable other items. A second answer is that it may be possible to choose from among health programs *without* placing a dollar value on human life; it may be sufficient to compare the marginal yield of different programs in terms of lives saved in order to determine the allocation of resources that yields the more significant social benefits.

PHYSICIANS OR OTHER MEDICAL CARE PROVIDERS?

But that is not the whole story. Even if we could make intelligent choices between medical care and other health-related programs, we would still be faced with a significant range of decisions concerning the best way to provide medical care — that is, the best way to spend the medical care dollar. One of the most important of these decisions, which will be discussed in Chapter 3, concerns the respective roles of physicians and such other medical care providers as physician assistants, nurses, clinicians, midwives, and family-health workers. A related set of decisions concerns the optimal mix between human inputs (whether physicians or others) and physical capital inputs, such as hospitals, X-ray equipment, and computers.

In short, if we are concerned with the best way to produce medical care, we must be aware that the solution to the problem requires more than medical expertise. It requires consideration of the relative prices, of various medical care inputs, and of their contribution (again at the margin) to health. The argument that these inputs must be used in some technologically defined proportions is soundly refuted by the evidence from other countries, where many health systems successfully utilize doctors, nurses, hospital facilities, and other health inputs in proportions that differ strikingly from those used in the United States.

HOW MUCH EQUALITY? AND HOW TO ACHIEVE IT?

One of the major choices any society must make is how far to go in equalizing the access of individuals to goods and services. Insofar as this is a question of social choice, one cannot look to economics for an answer. What economic analysis can do is provide some insights concerning why the distribution of income at any given time is what it is, what policies would alter it and at what cost, and what are the economic consequences of different distributions.

Assuming that some income equalization is desired, how is this to be accomplished? Shall only certain goods and services (say, medical care) be distributed equally, or should incomes be made more equal, leaving individuals to decide how they wish to adjust their spending to take account of their higher (or lower) income?

For any given amount of redistribution the welfare of all households is presumably greatest if there is a general tax on the income of some households and grants of income to others, rather than a tax on particular forms of spending or a subsidy for particular types of consumption. Common sense tells us that if a household is offered a choice of either a hundred dollars in cash or a hundred dollars' worth of health care, it ought to prefer the cash, because it can use the entire sum to buy more health care or health insurance (if that is what it wants) or, as is usually the case, increase consumption of many other commodities as well. By the same reasoning, if a household is offered a choice between paying an additional hundred dollars in income tax or doing without a hundred dollars' worth of health care, it will opt for the general tax on income, and then cut back spending on the goods and services that are, in its opinion, most dispensable.

Despite the obvious logic of the foregoing, many nonpoor seem more willing to support a reduction in inequality in the consumption of particular commodities (medical care is a conspicuous example) than toward a general redistribution of income. In England, for instance, everyone is eligible to use the National Health Service, and the great majority of the population gets all of its care from this tax-financed source. At the same time, there is considerable inequality in other aspects of British life, including education and income distribution in general.

Support for the notion that medical care ought to be available to all, regardless of ability to pay, is growing in the United States. There is, however, also growing recognition of marked disparities in housing, legal services, and other important goods and services. Whether these disparities should be attacked piecemeal or through a general redistribution of income is one of the most difficult questions facing the body politic. The pros and cons of this issue as it affects medical care will be discussed in Chapter 6.

TODAY OR TOMORROW

One of the most important choices every individual and every society has to make is between using existing resources to satisfy current desires or applying them to capital-creating activities in anticipation of future needs. Economists call the former *consumption* and the latter *investment.*

This broad concept of investment should not be confused with the narrow use of the term in financial transactions — e.g., the purchase of stock. Broadly speaking, investment takes place when a tree is planted, when a student goes to school, when you brush your teeth, as well as when you build a house, a factory, or a hospital. Any activity that can be expected to confer future benefits is a form of investment. (To be sure, sometimes a single activity — such as education — will have elements of consumption — that is, provide current satisfaction — along with those of investment.)

Such investment can be in both physical or human capital.* Thus health is a form of capital: health is wealth. Investment in health takes many forms. Immunization, annual checkups, exercise, and many other activities have current costs but may yield health benefits in the future. Medical education and medical research, both involving expenditures of billions of dollars annually, are prime examples of investment in the health field that results in the diversion of resources (physicians and other personnel) from meeting current needs in order to reap future rewards.

How far should we go in providing for tomorrow at the expense of today? As with all economic decisions, price plays a role here, too. Specifically, in making

*The development of the theory of human capital by Gary Becker, Jacob Mincer, T. W. Schultz, and others and its application in fields such as education and health is one of the great advances in economics in the past quarter-century.

decisions concerning health investments, we must somehow take into account the fact that people discount the future compared with the present. Using the concept of the special kind of price called *rate of interest* or *rate of return* answers that need.

No investment in health is undertaken unless the investor believes it will yield a satisfactory rate of return. Health professionals frequently despair over the failure of some people to invest in their own health; such behavior, they assert, is irrational. But this need not be the case. If a person discounts the future at a high rate, as evidenced by a willingness to pay 20 or 30 percent annual interest for consumer loans or installment credit, it would not be rational to make an investment in health that had an implicit return of only 15 percent.

It is abundantly clear that people differ in their attitudes toward the future; that is, they have different *rates of time discount.** The reasons for these differences are not known. They may be related to perceptions about how certain the future is, and they may depend upon how strongly rooted is one's sense of the past. Young children, for instance, characteristically live primarily in the present; they lack both a historical perspective and a vision of the future. Thus it is often difficult to get children to undertake some unpleasant task or to refrain from some pleasureable activity for the sake of a beneficial consequence five or ten years away. Some adults, too, set very little store in the future compared with the present; they have a very high rate of time discount.

Most health-related activities — smoking, exercise, diet, periodic checkups and so forth — have consequences which are realized only after long periods of time. One possible reason for the high correlation between an individual's health and length of schooling (see Chapter 2) is that attending to one's health and attending school are both aspects of investment in human capital. Thus the same person who has accumulated a great deal of human capital in the form of schooling may, for the same reasons, have made (or had made) substantial investments in health.

YOUR LIFE OR MINE?

Suppose a small private plane crashes in an isolated forest area and no one knows whether the pilot is dead or alive. How much of society's resources will be devoted to searching for the pilot? How much "should" be devoted to the search? If the pilot is a wealthy or prominent person, the search is likely to be longer and more thorough than if not. If the person is wealthy, then the respective family's command over private resources will make the difference; if the person is a prominent government official, it is likely that publicly owned resources will be utilized far more readily than if the person were unknown and poor.

Rate of time discount is a measure of how willing people are to incur present costs or defer present benefits in order to obtain some benefit in the future.

We see in this simple example one of the basic dilemmas of modern society. On the one hand, we believe that all people should be treated as equals, especially in matters of life or death. Against this we have what Raymond Aron calls the imperative "to produce as much as possible through mastery of the forces of nature,"[2] a venture requiring differentiation, hierarchy, and inevitably unequal treatment. The problem arises in all types of economic systems, and in all systems the response is likely to be similar.

If the family of a wealthy person wants to devote their wealth to the search for the missing person, thereby increasing the probability of survival, is there any reason why the rest of society should object? (If the family used their command over resources for some frivolous consumption, would anyone else be better off?) Suppose, however, that instead of a plane crash the threat of death came from an ordinarily fatal disease. Would the same answers apply? The capacity of medical science to intervene near the point of death is growing rapidly. Such interventions are often extremely costly and have a low probability of long-term success — but sometimes they work. Whose life should be saved? The wealthy person's? The senator's? Society cannot escape this problem any more than it can avoid facing the other choices we have discussed.

A related dilemma concerns the allocation of resources, either for research or care, among different diseases and conditions. The potential for social conflict here is high because the relative importance of different diseases is perceived differentially by groups according to their income level, race, age, location, and other characteristics.

A particularly striking example of this problem is sickle-cell anemia, a disease which in the United States affects primarily Blacks. Recently there has been a substantial increase in the amount of funds available for research on this as-yet-incurable disease, primarily as a result of the growing political strength of the Black community.

Many other diseases have a particularly high incidence among specific groups. Thus cigarette smokers have a much greater stake in research or services for lung cancer than do nonsmokers. And in the case of occupation-related diseases, the interests of workers and employers directly affected are much greater than those of the general public.

Economics cannot provide final answers to these difficult problems of social priorities, but it can help decision makers think more rationally about them. In allocating funds for medical research, for instance, economic reasoning can tell the decision maker what kind of information one ought to have and how to arrange that information so as to find the probable relative value of various courses of action.

Contrary to the opinion of many medical researchers, the criterion of "scientific merit" is not sufficient to form the basis for a rational allocation of medical research funds. Certainly decision makers should consider the relative importance the scientific community attaches to particular problems. But other kinds of information — such as the number of persons affected by a particular disease, the economic cost of the attendant morbidity* and mortality, and the cost of delivering preventive or therapeutic services if research is successful — should also be considered. The last item is particularly important when funding applied as opposed to basic research, because the development of a "cure" that is enormously expensive to implement probably has a low return and creates many serious social problems as well. For example, if a cure for cancer were discovered tomorrow but cost $150,000 per case to implement, the resulting controversies over the method of financing and the selection of cases to be cured might be so great as to make one view the cure as a mixed blessing.

THE JUNGLE OR THE ZOO?

One of the central choices of our time, in health as in other areas, is finding the proper balance between individual (personal) and collective (social) responsibility. If too much weight is given to the former, we come close to recreating the "jungle" — with all the freedom and all the insecurity that the jungle implies. On the other hand, emphasizing social responsibility can increase security, but it may be the security of the "zoo" — purchased at the expense of freedom. Over the centuries human beings have wrestled with this choice, and in different times and different places the emphasis has shifted markedly.

Nineteenth-century Western society idealized individual responsibility. This was particularly true in England and the United States, where a system of political economy was developed based on the teachings of Locke, Smith, Mill, and other advocates of personal freedom. As this system was superimposed on a religious foundation which exalted hard work and thrift, the result was an unprecedented acceleration in the rate of growth of material output. Each person's energies were bent to enhancing one's own welfare, secure in the knowledge that each individual and the respective family would enjoy the fruits of their efforts and in the conviction that they were obeying God's will.

That the system worked imperfectly goes without saying. That the outcome for some individuals was harsh and brutal has been recounted in innumerable novels, plays, histories, and sociological treatises. But when set against humankind's previous history, the material benefits and the accompanying relaxation of social, religious, and political rigidities were extraordinary.

By the beginning of this century, however, reactions to such uninhibited "progress" had arisen in most Western countries. Since then a variety of laws have been passed seeking to protect individuals from the most severe consequences of unbridled individualism. Laissez-faire is dead, and only a few mourn its passing. In fact, the attitude of many intellectuals and popular writers on political economy

*Morbidity is the extent of an illness in the population.

seems to have swung to the other extreme. In the 1920s R. H. Tawney, surveying the eighteenth- and nineteenth-century attitudes toward poverty, wrote that "the most curious feature in the whole discussion . . . was the resolute refusal to admit that society had any responsibility for the causes of distress."[3] Some future historian, in reviewing mid-twentieth-century social reform literature, may note an equally curious feature — a "resolute refusal" to admit that individuals have any responsibility for their own distress.

From the idealization of individual responsibility and the neglect of social responsibility we have gone, in some quarters, to the denial of individual responsibility and the idealization of social responsibility. The rejection of any sense of responsibility for one's fellow beings is inhuman, but the denial of any individual responsibility is also dehumanizing.

Moreover, with respect to health such a view runs contrary to common sense. As Henry Sigerist, an ardent advocate of socialized medicine and other expressions of social responsibility, has observed: "The state can protect society very effectively against a great many dangers, but the cultivation of health, which requires a definite mode of living, remains, to a large extent, an individual matter."[4] Most of us know this is true from personal experience. As long as we believe that we have some control over our own choices, we will reject theories that assume that "society" is always the villain.

A great deal of what has been written recently about "the right to health" is very misleading. It suggests that society has a supply of "health" stored away which it can give to individuals and that it is only the niggardliness of the Administration or the ineptness of Congress or the selfishness of physicians that prevents this from happening. Such a view ignores the truth of Douglas Colman's observation that "positive health is not something that one human can hand to or require of another. Positive health can be achieved only through intelligent effort on the part of each individual. Absent that effort, health professionals can only insulate the individual from the more catastrophic results of his ignorance, self-indulgence, or lack of motivation."[5] The notion that we can spend our way to better health is a vast oversimplification. At present there is very little that medical care can do for a lung that has been overinflated by smoking, or for a liver that has been scarred by too much alcohol, or for a skull that has been crushed in a motor accident.

The assertion that *medical care* is (or should be) a "right" is more plausible. In a sense medical care is to health what schooling is to wisdom. No society can truthfully promise to make everyone wise, but society can make schooling freely available; it can even make it compulsory. Many countries have taken a similar position with respect to medical care, although the compulsory aspects are sharply limited. Our government could, if it wished to, come close to assuring access to medical care for all persons. But no government now or in the foreseeable future can assure health to every individual.

Because utilization of medical care is voluntary, the mere availability of a service does not guarantee its use. The discovery of polio vaccine was rightly hailed as a significant medical advance, but in recent years there has been a sharp drop in the proportion of children receiving such vaccinations. At present, probably one-third of the children between 1 and 4 years of age are not adequately protected. The problem is particularly acute in poverty areas of major cities, where as many as half the children probably are without full protection against polio. There are undoubtedly many difficulties facing poor families that make it more difficult for them to bring their children to be vaccinated, but the service itself is available in most cities.

Another example of a gap between availability and utilization comes from a study of dental services covered by group health insurance. The study reported that white-collar workers and their families used significantly more preventive services than their blue-collar counterparts even though the insurance policy provided full coverage for all participants. The only dental service used more frequently by blue-collar families was tooth extraction — a procedure which is usually a consequence of failure to use preventive services, such as repair of caries.

If people have a *right* to care, do they also have an *obligation* to use it?
This complex question will assume greater significance as the collective provision of care increases. In our zeal to raise health levels, however, we must be wary of impinging on other valuable "rights," including the right to be left alone. Strict control over a person's behavior might well result in increased life expectancy, but a well-run zoo is still a zoo and not a worthy model for humankind.

As we attempt to formulate responsible policy for health and medical care, we should strive for the balance advocated by Rabbi Hillel more than two thousand years ago when he said, "If I am not for myself, who will be for me, but if I am for myself alone, what am I?"

The preceding discussion of the choices that face our society helps to put the major problems of health and medical care in proper perspective. These problems, as perceived by the public, are high cost, poor access, and inadequate health levels. In order to attack them intelligently, we must recognize the scarcity of resources and the need to allocate them as efficiently as possible. We must recognize that we can't have everything. In short, we need to adopt an economic point of view.

The discussion of choices also reveals some of the limits of economics in dealing with the most fundamental questions of health and medical care. These questions are ultimately ones of value: What value do we put on saving a life? on reducing pain? on relieving anxiety? How do these values change when the life at stake is a relative's? a neighbor's? a stranger's?

Nearly all human behavior is guided by values. Given the values, together with information about the relationship between technological means and ends, about inputs and constraints (resources, time, money), economics shows how these values can be maximized. To the extent that individual behavior attempts to maximize values, economic theory also possesses significant power to predict behavior. If and when values change and these changes are not taken into account, however, economics loses a good deal of its predictive power. The most difficult part of the problem is that values may change partly as a result of the economic process itself.

According to one well-known definition, "economics is the science of means, not of ends": it can explain how market prices are determined, but not how basic values are formed; it can tell us the consequences of various alternatives, but it cannot make the choice for us. These limitations will be with us always, for economics can never replace morals or ethics.

Supplementary Reading

Please see "Major Concepts of Health Care Economics" and "Major Trends in the U.S. Health Economy Since 1950" in Part 2.

CHAPTER 2

Who Shall Live?

> Who shall live and who shall die, who shall
> fulfill his days and who shall die before his
> time... .
>
> Yom Kippur (Day of Atonement)
> prayer book

Good health and long life have traditionally been among the most prized goals of humankind. In every age and in every land there have been significant efforts to postpone death, whether through sacred dance and song, the imbibing of magic potions, or the application of the most modern medical techniques.

Despite these efforts, for most of human history life was short and uncertain. It depended primarily upon such basic economic conditions as adequate supplies of food, water, and shelter. Healers of all kinds were abundant, but apart from the sympathy and psychological support that they may have provided, it is doubtful that they did more good than harm. Historians of medicine now mostly agree that it was not until well into the twentieth century that the average patient had better than a fifty-fifty chance of being helped by the average physician.

Today, at least in developed countries, the situation is markedly different. First, there is a core of medical knowledge that contributes greatly to life expectancy. This knowledge is widely diffused throughout the United States, Europe, Japan, and Oceania and is even reducing mortality in less developed countries, including some with very low standards of living. That portion of medicine which is most dramatically effective, such as vaccines and antiinfectious drugs, is relatively simple and inexpensive to administer. But once basic levels of medical sophistication, personnel, and facilities become available, additional inputs of medical care do not have much effect. In other words, the total contribution of modern medical care to life expectancy is large, but over the considerable range of variation in the quantity of care observed in developed countries, the marginal contribution is small.

A second profound change is the disappearance of the traditional relationship between life expectancy and per capita income. As with medical care, a certain minimum level of income is important, but beyond that there is little correlation between mortality and income across and within industrialized countries.

These themes comprise the focus of this chapter, which also highlights the importance of "life-style" and personal behavior as major determinants of "who shall live."

The First Year of Life

The human infant is an exceptionally vulnerable creature. It comes into the world with a precarious hold on life; unassisted, it cannot live for more than a week. This extreme dependency on others persists much longer in humans than in any other species and is the major reason why human beings require an elaborate social structure.

Consideration of the complex support mechanisms required for human survival reveals the fallacies in the arguments of extreme libertarians and romantics. The former assume that people are autonomous, beholden to no one, answerable to no one, capable of rationally determining their own fate on the basis of contractual relationships with other autonomous souls. In fact, each of us owes our very life to others. Without the care given by family or friends, or provided by the church or state, we would not be alive to propound theories of human independence.

Rousseau and other romantics have viewed humans as being born into a free and golden future only to be shackled by family and society. The truth is that throughout history most human beings have been born into a promise of early death. The more "simple" the environment, the more certain was it that the promise would be fulfilled. Even when the infant's mother survived childbirth (until this century the risk of maternal mortality was not small) and was willing to care for her child as best she could, prospects for its survival were not good.

Under primitive conditions it is not unusual for one out of every two newborns to die before the age of one; for many families the survival rate is much worse. Enrico Caruso, the great Italian tenor, was the eighteenth child born to his poor Neapolitan parents but the first to survive beyond infancy. According to one estimate, the infant mortality rate (the number of deaths in the first year of life per 1,000 live births) for Europe's *ruling families* was over 200 in the sixteenth and seventeenth centuries.[1] The rate for families of lesser means must have been appreciably higher, for, as indicated below, chances for survival improved markedly with increases in living standards.

By the nineteenth century, infant mortality for Europe's ruling families was down to 70. But in New York City the rate for the general population was still as high as 140 per 1,000 live births in 1900. With rising living standards the chances of infant survival began to improve markedly. Between 1900 and 1930 the infant mortality in the United States fell at an annual rate of 2.5 percent to 65 per 1,000, and similar declines were experienced by all other countries undergoing rapid economic development. Most of this decline was the result of a sharp reduction in deaths from what physicians call the "pneumonia-diarrhea" complex.* In New York City infant mortality from this cause fell from 75 in 1900 to about 17 in 1930.

It is important to realize that medical care played almost no role in this decline. While we do not know the precise causes, it is believed that rising living standards, the spread of literacy and education, and a substantial fall in the birth rate all played a part. Some writers also give credit to chlorination of the water supply and the pasteurization of milk, but there is considerable debate about the quantitative importance of these measures. The "pneumonia-diarrhea" complex is still a major killer of infants on some American Indian reservations, and one well-studied attempt to bring all the skills of medicine to bear on this problem was, on the whole, unsuccessful.[2]

The mid-1930s saw the introduction of sulfonamide, the first of the great antimicrobial drugs. During the fifteen years that followed, many other potent antiinfectious drugs were discovered, and the rate of decline in infant mortality improved substantially. Between 1935 and 1950 the infant death rate fell by 4.3 percent annually, an appreciable acceleration over the decline of preceding decades. During this period both medical advances and rising living standards contributed to the reduction in infant deaths.

By 1950, about 70 percent of all infant deaths were occurring in the first month after birth, compared to only 40 percent in 1900. Such "neonatal" deaths, which are usually related to prematurity, congenital malformations, and problems associated with delivery, have proved less responsive to the growth of real income and to medical advances. It is not surprising, therefore, that beginning about 1950 there was a marked deterioration in the rate of decline of infant mortality. Between 1950 and 1965, the average annual decline was only 1.1 percent. During that period there was a great deal of talk about having reached some minimum level below which it would be very difficult to go.

Then, fairly suddenly, infant mortality began to drop again sharply, and since 1965 the rate of decline has been over 4 percent annually. By 1971 the U.S. rate had fallen to 19.2. The reasons for this marked improvement are not known. One possible explanation is that there was a substantial decrease in "unwanted" births after 1965 as a result of improved contraception and more liberal abortion laws.

---

*A common cause of death among infants living in poor, unsanitary conditions is internal infection leading to diarrhea which so weakens the infant that it contracts fatal pneumonia.

Indeed, the U.S. birth rate fell from 19.4 per 1,000 population in 1965 to 15.1 in 1973. The birth rate for births of fourth order or higher (i.e., those in which the mother has had at least three other children), which present a greater risk, fell by 50 percent. There can be little doubt that a "wanted" child will receive better care, both during pregnancy and after birth, than one that is "unwanted."

Furthermore, beginning in the late 1960s more was done to combat infant deaths by extending maternal and infant care services to families that had not previously been as well served. In some particular settings substantial reductions in infant deaths were achieved through the use of intensive-care units for premature babies, which have greatest risk. How important such additional medical care was in affecting the overall trend, however, is not known.

PREMATURITY

Numerous studies of infant mortality have shown that low-birth-weight babies (defined as under 5½ pounds) face considerably higher risk of death than those of normal weight. One comprehensive report issued by the federal government's National Center for Health Statistics states that "such infants have thirty times the risk of dying in the first four weeks of life compared with infants weighing more than 2500 grams [5½ pounds] at birth."[3] The correlation between low birth weight and post-neonatal deaths is much weaker, but according to one authority, "the premature infant not only has a poorer chance of surviving, ... but if he does survive he has a higher risk of having a handicapping condition."[4]

We know surprisingly little about the specific reasons for short gestation (premature delivery) or low birth weight. The physical condition of the mother is undoubtedly a major factor, and this in turn is probably related to her diet, to whether she smokes or not, and to other environmental influences. Some of the variables found to be associated with low birth weight and infant mortality in general are income, schooling, race, and prenatal care.

INCOME

Traditionally, as income goes up, infant mortality goes down. In recent years, however, this relationship has become weaker for two primary reasons. First, the relationship was always much stronger for post-neonatal deaths (those occurring in the first year but after the first month) than for neonatal deaths. But today, as noted earlier, infant mortality in developed countries is concentrated in the first month.

A second reason is that once income rises to a level that assures adequate nutrition, housing, water, and waste disposal, further increases in income have much less significance for life expectancy. Most American families have passed that minimum level. A study published in 1972 and based on 1964–1966 data showed appreciable declines in White infant death rates as family income rose from under

$3,000 to the $5,000–7,000 range. Above that income level, however, there was no further decline with rising income.[5]

A third possible reason for a weakening of this relationship is a wider diffusion of medical care throughout the population. The extent of this diffusion and its effectiveness are, however, open to question. It is relevant to note that large differences in infant mortality among socioeconomic classes in England and Scotland persist despite the existence of free national health services available to all segments of the population.

SCHOOLING

Numerous health studies have shown that length of schooling is one of the most important correlates of health. This is true regardless of the measure of health (mortality, morbidity, or days lost from work) and regardless of whether the data are for individuals or population averages. Infant mortality also conforms to this pattern: in the United States, infants born to White mothers with eight years of schooling or less have almost double the mortality rate of those born to mothers with twelve or more years of schooling. (The correlation with length of father's schooling is also very strong.)

There is, of course, also a very strong correlation between schooling and income, making it difficult to estimate the separate effects of each. There does, however, seem to be some independent contribution to infant health both from schooling and from income. Among *adults* the relationship between schooling and health is much stronger, although, as we shall see in the next section, the effect of income is weak.

RACE

If one wanted a single simple index of the cumulative effects of hundreds of years of prejudice and oppression, the fact that in the United States Black infant mortality is almost double the White rate would serve as well as any.

Some investigators believe that this difference can be explained mostly or entirely by a few socioeconomic variables; others report data that refute this view. It does seem clear that the excess of Black over White infant death rates is greater than can be explained by *current* differences in income or schooling. As an illustration, *Black* infant mortality in New York and California is two-thirds greater than *White* infant mortality in Arkansas and South Carolina, although income and schooling levels are comparable.

Low birth weight is the major factor in Black infant mortality (as it is in White). Why so many Black infants should be born weighing under 5½ pounds is not known. Diet, rest, and other aspects of care during pregnancy are probably important. It may also be true that the deprived conditions of many Black families a generation ago are still taking their toll today. Scientists have shown with animal experiments that nutritional deprivation of females in infancy can affect their subsequent reproductive performance, even when they are provided with adequate diet as adults. Sir Dugald Baird, Regius Professor of Obstetrics and Gynecology at the University of Aberdeen, Scotland, has suggested that this mechanism may also be at work among humans. Finding that infant deaths from malformation of the central nervous system rose sharply in 1946 in first births to women in the semiskilled and unskilled occupational classes, he concluded that "the increase in the death rate could not be traced to any factor operating during the mother's pregnancy, but seemed to be related to the year in which the mother was born. For example, the rates were highest in women born between 1928 and 1936, the years during which the economic depression was at its worst."[6]

Although infant mortality for American Blacks has declined over time, just as it has for American Whites, the relative differential has not changed much. This is somewhat surprising because, given the diminishing importance of income on infant mortality as income rises, one might have expected the infant mortality gap to narrow even though relative income differentials have remained about the same. One possibility is that reported Black infant death rates for earlier decades were understated because many deaths went unreported. Inequality of access to medical care is also frequently cited as a reason for the Black–White differential in infant mortality. But this inequality is probably less now than in earlier decades, and, in any case, the role of medical care in determining the outcome of pregnancy is a subject of considerable controversy.

MEDICAL CARE

Medical care enthusiasts insist that every pregnant woman should consult an obstetrical specialist early in her pregnancy, should continue to visit that specialist frequently, and should be delivered in a hospital with a full range of attending health personnel and elaborate facilities. Skeptics like to point out that in the Netherlands, where a substantial proportion of all births occur at home under the supervision of a midwife, the infant mortality rate is one of the lowest in the world. The Dutch example suggests that *how* medical care is used may be more important than *how much* is used.

The strongest evidence that medical care does have a significant effect on infant mortality appears in a study published by the Institute of Medicine of the National Academy of Sciences. All deliveries in New York City during 1968 were classified according to ethnic group, social and medical risk, and adequacy of medical care during pregnancy and delivery. The study found that within each ethnic-risk category, infant mortality was much lower for the children born to mothers who had adequate care. If the infant mortality rate of children born to mothers with *inadequate* care could have been reduced to the rate of the adequate-care groups, the overall rate for the city would have been 18.4 instead of 21.9 per 1,000 live births.[7] This method of calculation surely overstates the contribution of medical care by assuming that within a given ethnic-risk category *all* of the difference in infant mortality between groups getting different levels of care was in fact due to the care. Furthermore, even a reduction to 18.4 would have left infant mortality in New York City considerably above the rates recorded in Scandinavia and the Netherlands for that same year. Factors other than medical care are clearly of major significance.

Variation in infant mortality rates among various states in this country does not reflect any significant correlation between rate and the number of physicians per capita after account is taken of differences in income, schooling, and similar variables.[8] Such studies, however, deal only with average results. Medical care programs aimed at groups of particularly high risk — very young girls, women of low socioeconomic status, and the like — have in recent years been able to show substantial reductions in neonatal mortality. Therein may lie an important clue to the role of medical care. For very risky pregnancies, the quantity and quality of care available may be critical; for pregnancies that present little risk (that is, among well-educated, well-fed mothers, neither very young nor very old) the quantity and quality of care may be of minor importance, except insofar as poor care can be worse than none at all.

The possibility that medical care can do harm as well as good is a real and growing one. As the tools of medical intervention — drugs, surgery, radiotherapy, and the like — become more powerful, the risks of iatrogenic disease (ill health arising out of the medical care process itself) increase. For example, two decades ago it was standard procedure in the best hospitals to administer oxygen to low-birth-weight babies. It is now believed that this practice was responsible for considerable retrolental fibroplasia, which leads to blindness.

It is easy to assemble a catalog of horror stories about misdirected medical efforts, but this, too, can be misleading. It is obvious that as knowledge grows in medicine, some of the presently accepted therapies will be found to be useless or even harmful. It is also obvious that mistakes are made in every field and by every profession. What is required is some sense of balance so that the contribution of medical care is not oversold and so that both patient and provider realize the wisdom in the ancient warning to physicians, "Do no harm."

INTERNATIONAL COMPARISONS

What light, if any, do the preceding considerations throw on the large international differences in infant mortality that presently exist? If we compare developed countries with less developed ones, they explain a great deal. But if we confine our attention to differences among developed countries, they don't provide much help.

The lowest rates, averaging about 13 per 1,000 in 1970, are found in the Netherlands, Scandinavia, Australia, New Zealand, and Japan, all countries having relatively high levels of income and schooling. Yet in the United States, which has even higher income and education levels, the rate in 1970 was almost 20 per 1,000. The rate for U.S. Whites was 17.4; and for Whites in North Dakota, the most favorable state in the country, but certainly not the wealthiest, the rate was 14.

In comparison with *large* European countries, however, the United States does not fare so badly: in 1970 the infant mortality in Italy was 29.2, in West Germany 23.6, in the United Kingdom 18.3, and in France 15.1. Our neighbor, Canada, had almost exactly the same rate as we did, and highly industrialized Belgium and Luxembourg were slightly worse off.

It has been popular to use international comparisons in infant mortality as a stick with which to beat the American medical profession. Some of this criticism has been constructive. It has shattered the smug and incorrect assumption that "Americans have the best health in the world." It has also helped to dramatize gross disparities within this country. Perhaps most important, it has forced some leaders in medicine to begin focusing on health *outcomes* as the criteria of "quality," instead of preoccupying themselves with credentials, expensive equipment, and other ingredients of the *process* of care.

If one examines the data closely, however, the claim that the wide disparities between the U.S. infant mortality rate and rates elsewhere are primarily attributable to deficiencies in American medicine becomes unpersuasive. Many of these differences are of long standing. The U.S. rate was substantially higher than the rate in the Netherlands or New Zealand, for example, long before medical care could have made much difference either way. Even the presence of free national health services does not guarantee low rates, as the United Kingdom data indicate.

In the final analysis, we must recognize the critical importance of the mother — the care she takes of herself during pregnancy and the care she provides for the child after birth. Effective family planning — that is, the bearing of children when and in the number that the parents want — is surely also important in achieving low infant mortality. Just how religion, culture, the political, economic, and social structure, medical care, and other forces combine to affect the outcome of pregnancy remains to be determined.

INFANT HEALTH

Mere survival is not, of course, everything. We want to raise children who will be equipped mentally and physically to contribute to the world's work and to share in the pleasures life has to offer. Their capacity to do this as adults may be dramatically affected by what happens to them during the first year of life. As Dr. Walsh McDermott notes: "We are beginning to get a solid scientific base for the concept that mental capacity and the capability to be educated can be permanently impaired by early infancy."[9]

There is a widespread belief that reductions in infant and child mortality keep alive persons with "weak constitutions" or other health impairments, thus increasing the health problems and death rates of the population when they become adults. A contrary point of view, however, should be considered. It can be argued that the same forces, socioeconomic and medical, that reduce mortality among infants and children also strengthen the health of those who would have survived anyway, albeit marginally. Mortality can be viewed as one end of a distribution of health conditions, and reductions in mortality can be viewed as part of a more general process which shifts the entire distribution in the direction of better health.

A long-term British study of more than seventeen thousand births has shown that not only do low-birth-weight babies have less chance of surviving, but those that do survive are more likely to have other problems (behavior, learning ability, etc.) by the time they reach school age. Thus, the same measures that offer the most promise for lowering infant mortality (improved nutrition, reduction in cigarette smoking, better timing and spacing of births, and the like) will probably raise rather than lower the quality of life for those who survive.

One thing is clear. The decrease in U.S. infant mortality over the years has *not* resulted in higher death rates among children or adults. Nor does the lower infant mortality in Scandinavia mean that death rates there exceed those of the United States at subsequent ages. The next section provides a closer look at the factors associated with adult mortality.

Three Score and Ten

The days of our years are three score years and ten.

Psalms 90 : 10

According to the Bible, the normal life span for humans was 70 years. This was not an absolute upper limit: the psalmist did hold out the possibility of 80 years "by reason of strength." Neither was this life expectancy in the technical sense of the term (the average number of years lived by all persons born at a particular time). Indeed, life expectancy in the biblical era was probably less than 35 years. A more plausible interpretation is that this was the "expected" life span in the sense that people could not expect to live beyond that age, assuming they were among the fortunate ones who survived the perils of infancy, childhood, and young adulthood.

In this sense the estimate has remarkable force, even today. In the United States more than half of those who reach the age of 70 will die during the subsequent decade, and after 80 the death rate becomes very high indeed. The great increase in life expectancy that has occurred in developed countries over the past two hundred years has been the result primarily of reductions in death rates at early ages, not in the lengthening of the "normal" life span.

Life expectancy is now almost exactly 70 years in the United States, and slightly higher in some other countries. Comparison of life tables from various countries at various times suggests that as life expectancy rises from 35 to 70, about four-fifths of the increase is contributed by reductions in death rates under 70 and only one-fifth comes from reductions in death rates at age 70 or above.

We have already reviewed the significant reductions in infant mortality that have been achieved in this century. The fall in death rates for children over the age of 1 year has been even more impressive. For ages 1 through 4 the decline has been almost 5 percent annually; this means that on the average the death rate for this group has been halved every 15 years since 1900. For the 5-to-14-year-old group the annual decrease has been at about 3.5 percent, more rapid than the annual 3 percent decline in infant mortality over the same period.

The decrease in the child death rate has been particularly striking since the 1930s as the result of advances in medicine. One by one the dread diseases of childhood — pneumonia, influenza, diphtheria, typhoid fever, polio, and so on — have succumbed to immunization or powerful new drug therapies. The reduction in parental grief and fear brought about by rising living standards and medical advances surely stands as one of the greatest achievements of industrial society. Today, the risk of death in all the years between 1 and 20 combined is appreciably less than in the first year alone!

Although most Americans can now expect to reach the age of 70, about four in ten do not. An examination of the causes of death in adolescents and young adults (ages 15–24), in early middle age (35–44), and in late middle age (55–64) will give us a clearer understanding of the role economic and social factors play in early death and what medical care can and cannot do to prevent them.

YOUTH: AGES 15–24

Adolescents and young adults are on the whole extremely healthy. Their strength, energy, capacity to go without sleep, withstand the elements, and shake off minor infirmities are the envy of their elders. In the United States their chances of dying from "normal" diseases are very small indeed. Unfortunately, their overall probability of death is not that small, especially for males. Because the sex differential in mortality is so large in the United States, it is given an extended discussion later in this chapter. For the moment we shall concentrate on *male* deaths, highlighting the differences associated with age and color.*

Suppose we consider 100,000 American males age 15. The following figures show how many will die from selected causes and all causes before they reach the age of 25, assuming that the latest available death rates (1968) continue unchanged.†

Expected Number of Deaths per 100,000
from Ages 15 through 24

CAUSE OF DEATH	WHITE MALES	NON-WHITE MALES
Motor accidents	807	661
Other accidents	310	545
Suicide	113	82
Neoplasms	103	82
Homicide	75	771
Influenza and pneumonia	29	58
Heart diseases	28	69
All causes	1,690	2,777

The most striking aspect of these data is the tremendous loss of life from accidents, especially motor accidents. Of every one hundred thousand American males age 15, about 1,100 will lose their lives in accidents before reaching 25; more than half of those deaths will involve automobiles. "Epidemic" is almost too weak a word to describe this situation; when polio was at its worst, the death rate from that disease among males ages 15 to 24 was less than one twentieth as high. To be sure, polio causes illness as well as death, but the disabilities and impairments resulting from auto accidents also far exceed the number killed.

Also striking is the fact that *homicide* is the leading cause of death among young Black males; indeed, it continues to be a significant cause of death right up through middle age. Thus if you are a 15-year-old Black American

*The data are for Whites and non-Whites; Blacks account for about 95 percent of non-White male deaths at the ages discussed in this chapter.

†All the United States mortality statistics presented in the following pages are calculated from data in Department of Health, Education, and Welfare *Vital Statistics of the United States*, Vol. 2, *Mortality*, Part A, Table 1–9: Death Rates for 69 Selected Causes, by 10-Year Age Groups, Color, and Sex (Washington, DC: Government Printing Office, 1968).

male, your chances of being a homicide victim sometime before you reach 55 are thirty out of a thousand — more than triple the risk of your dying from tuberculosis.

Among young White males, suicide claims almost as many victims as do neoplasms (cancer and related illnesses) and heart disease combined. When one considers that many auto deaths might well be classified as suicide, it is apparent that the self-destructiveness of young American males is a major health problem today. The suicide rate for young Black males is lower than for Whites, but has been increasing at a faster rate.

Accidents, suicide, homicide — deaths from violence in one form or another account for *three out of every four* male deaths in this age group. Twenty years ago, the overall death rate among this age group was 15 percent lower, and the rate for violent deaths was 40 percent lower! The increase since then can hardly be attributed to a deterioration in medical care. On the contrary, the treatment of trauma is an area of medicine that has seen particularly significant advances, and there are undoubtedly many victims of violence being saved today who would have died two decades ago.

Numerous theories have been advanced to explain the increase in violent deaths among the young — affluence, the Vietnam war, the decline in religious belief, overly permissive parents, and so on — but the only thing we can be certain of is the increase itself. The suspicion also exists that the self-destructiveness of the young is a symptom of more widespread problems in society at large.

Among all U.S. males, deaths from accidents, suicide, and homicide account for one in every ten. Moreover, the cost to society of these deaths is relatively much greater than those due to other causes because so many of them involve men who had many productive years ahead of them. One frequently used measure of the economic cost of premature death is based on the earnings a man would have realized had he lived, discounted to take account of the fact that a dollar in hand is worth more than the expectation of a dollar sometime in the future. When deaths are weighted in this way, we find that violent deaths accounted for about 25 percent of the economic cost of all male deaths in 1968, compared to only 17 percent of the cost in 1960.

THE PRIME OF LIFE: AGES 35–44

By the time a White male American reaches 35 years of age, his chances of dying in a motor accident are less than half of what they were when he was 20. As we can see from the following figures, however, deaths from violence continue to take a heavy toll, still accounting for almost three out of every ten deaths.

Diseases of the heart become the number-one cause of death at about age 35 and continue to hold that position from then on. Between ages 35 and 45 approximately one White male out of every hundred dies of a heart attack or related disease. Among Black males the figure is approximately two out of a hundred. Neoplasms, especially lung cancer, also become significant among American males at age 35. Cirrhosis of the liver, which is usually attributable to alcoholism, is another major cause of death, exceeding even lung cancer in number of fatal victims. The *total* impact of smoking and drinking on health is thus apparently very great: in addition to the toll from lung cancer and cirrhosis, there are such other effects as the contribution of cigarettes to heart disease and of alcohol to motor accidents.

The differential between non-Whites and Whites at ages 35–44 is very pronounced; however the rates for non-Whites may contain some upward bias because of substantial underenumeration of Black males of this age in the Census of Population. The numerator in the death rate ratio (the number of deaths) is more accurately measured than the denominator (the population).

LATE MIDDLE AGE: AGES 55–64

By age 55 the risks of death of American males increase appreciably, as can be seen in the following figures:

*Expected Number of Deaths per 100,000
from Ages 35 through 44*

CAUSE OF DEATH	WHITE MALES	NON-WHITE MALES
Heart diseases	999	1,831
Neoplasms	507	803
(lung cancer)	(146)	(285)
Motor accidents	351	596
Other accidents	321	787
Suicide	232	126
Cirrhosis of liver	188	557
Homicide	98	1,146
Influenza and pneumonia	79	422
All causes	3,458	9,203

The chances of dying between ages 55 and 64 are much greater than during the entire period between ages 15 and 55. The major reason is the sharp increase in the chances of succumbing to a heart attack. For White males the death rate from this cause is ten times what it is at ages 35–44, and it accounts for half of all deaths in this age group. The death rate from lung cancer is also more than ten times greater than at ages 35–44. In both cases, behavior *earlier in life* may have started the fatal process, the consequences of which are realized only after several decades.

One unusual difference between Whites and non-Whites that is worth noting concerns their respective rates of suicide: the White rate is higher for all three age groups discussed here and the differential tends to increase with age. Such statistics seem to contradict the belief that low income and related problems are major causes of suicide; they suggest that an individual's perception of what constitutes low income may depend as much, or more, on expectations as on absolute dollar amounts.

COMPARISON WITH SWEDEN

Some insight into the health problems of American males can be obtained by comparing the White American death rates already presented with comparable rates for Swedish males, whose rates are among the most favorable in the world.*

Expected Number of Deaths per 100,000
from Ages 55 through 64

CAUSE OF DEATH	WHITE MALES	NON-WHITE MALES
Heart diseases	9,940	11,679
Neoplasms	4,697	6,484
(lung cancer)	(1,848)	(2,148)
Cerebrovascular disease	1,196	3,519
Cirrhosis of liver	645	677
Other accidents	508	945
Influenza and pneumonia	505	1,210
Motor accidents	382	628
Suicide	348	120
Homicide	62	508
All causes	21,902	32,607

At ages 15–24, the U.S. rate is 62 percent higher than the Swedish rate; thus the differential between White American males and Swedish males is as large as that between U.S. non-Whites and Whites. The major reason for the White American-Swedish differential is the high rate of violent deaths in the United States. Violent deaths show a differential of 83 percent, while the excess of White American over Swedish nonviolent deaths is only 16 percent. The motor accident death rate for White American males, for example, is about two-and-one-half times that for Swedish males.

*The Swedish mortality statistics presented in the following pages are calculated from data in United Nations, *Demographic Yearbook 1967* (New York: United Nations, 1968), Tables 5 and 25.

Expected Number of Deaths per 100,000
Swedish Males at Various Ages

CAUSE OF DEATH	15–24	35–44	55–64
Heart diseases	22	369	5,293
Neoplasms	110	343	3,159
Cerebrovascular disease	6	76	950
Cirrhosis of liver	—	50	204
Other accidents	228	287	426
Influenza and pneumonia	25	30	310
Motor accidents	335	197	285
Suicide	140	427	520
Homicide	9	4	9
All causes	1,045	2,286	13,410

In the 35–44 age group the pattern changes. The overall differential (White American-Swedish) is still 51 percent, but deaths from violence are only 10 percent greater in the United States. The differential at early middle age is because deaths from heart disease at this point are almost three times as likely in the United States as in Sweden. The excess of deaths from this cause alone accounts for well over half of the total excess in the White male American death rate in the age group. By ages 55–64 the U.S.-Swedish differential is 63 percent, and the U.S. rate for heart diseases is still double the Swedish rate.

A reasonable inference from these comparisons is that the huge mortality difference between the two countries is not connected to the quantity or quality of medical care. At younger ages the difference is mostly attributable to violent deaths, and at middle age the excess is primarily due to heart disease, which is probably related to diet, exercise, smoking, and stress. Given our present state of knowledge, even the most lavish use of medical care probably would not bring the U.S. rate more than a small step closer to the Swedish rate. Of course, as our knowledge grows this situation could change. For instance, some progress is being made in sorting out genetic factors that increase one's likelihood of suffering a heart attack, research that could lead to early detection of susceptible persons and possibly to preventive measures that would reduce their risk. At present, however, the greatest potential for reducing coronary disease, cancer, and the other major killers still lies in altering personal behavior.

THE CORRELATION WITH SCHOOLING

One of the most striking findings of recent research on the socioeconomic determinants of health in the United States is the strong positive correlation between health and length of schooling. This result holds for several types of health indexes ranging from mortality rates to self-evaluation of health status and for comparisons of individuals or populations such as cities or states. It also holds after allowing for the effects of such other variables as income, intelligence, and parents' schooling.

This relationship *may* reflect a chain of causality that begins with good health and results in more schooling. In the most detailed investigation yet undertaken of this subject, however, Michael Grossman has shown that the reverse hypothesis — that more schooling leads to better health — stands up well under a number of critical tests.[10] One of Grossman's most interesting findings concerns the relationship between schooling and premature death. Suppose you were studying, as he was, a group of White men in their thirties and you wanted to predict which ones would die in the next ten years. According to his results, educational attainment would have more predictive power that any other socioeconomic variable — including income and intelligence, two variables that are usually highly correlated with schooling.

Of course, neither Grossman nor anyone else is certain *why* or *how* schooling affects health. It may result in more sensible living habits; it may contribute to more effective use of medical care; or it may help people absorb new information about health and medical care more rapidly.

One possibility is that the completion of formal schooling increases self-confidence and thus reduces the stress associated with many social and work situations. Among business executives, for instance, it would not be surprising if those who work their way up from blue-collar positions are more prone to heart disease and ulcers than those who enter the executive suite via graduate schools of business. Another possibility is that both schooling and health are aspects of investment in human capital. Differences among individuals and their families in willingness and ability to make such investments may help explain the observed relationship.

So far all research on the relationship between health and schooling has utilized retrospective statistical analysis and thus is lacking in the precision and definitiveness of controlled experiments. Such research has nevertheless suggested an important connection between an individual's behavior and health. Additional support for this view emerges from a consideration of male–female differences in mortality, the subject of the following section.

The "Weaker" Sex

Judged by that harshest and in some sense most significant of all tests, the ability to survive, females are clearly much stronger than males. In all developed countries and at all ages the female death rate is appreciably below that of the male. This fact has significant economic and social consequences. For instance, by age 60, when female life expectancy is still 20 years, more than one out of five American females is a widow and another 10 percent are single or divorced with very little prospect of remarriage. An exploration of the extent of and variations in the sex differential in mortality rates at different ages and for different populations provides new insights into some current major health problems in the United States and their relation to economic and social factors.

THE AGE PATTERN

The excess of male over female deaths varies considerably with age. The differential is manifest even before birth, with the fetal death rate of males running about 10 percent above the rate of females. Since this differential emerges before the child's sex is known, there are clearly some biological differences at work in addition to the cultural and social factors that come into play after birth.

In the United States infant mortality among males is about one-third higher than for females, and throughout childhood the excess is in the range of one-third to one-half (see Figure 1). At age 15 the differential starts to rise sharply. Males between 15 and 24 have a death rate which is almost triple that of females, largely because of the high rate of violent deaths among males that we previously described. Indeed, if we exclude violent deaths, the differential is only 40 percent — about the same range as for infants and children.

The differential begins to fall during the late 20s and continues to do so until about age 40, at which point the male death rate is about 75 percent above the female rate. Then it begins to rise again, so that by age 60 the probability of death for males is more than double that for females. At this age the high incidence of heart disease in males is the principal cause of the differential. The male death rate from heart diseases is more than triple the female rate, while the differential for all other causes is only about 50 percent.

In old age the differential declines again, but even at ages 80–84 the male death rate is 25 percent above the female rate. Thus, over the entire life span the average differential is more than 75 percent, with the smallest differences at very young and very old ages and the biggest differences in the early 20s and early 60s.

VARIATIONS IN THE PATTERN

Although the basic shape of the age pattern is similar for most populations, there are some significant differences within the United States and between the United States and other countries that are worthy of attention. At young ages the differential of one-third to one-half is fairly constant for all developed countries and for different parts of the United States, suggesting that some inherent biological difference is the primary explanation. After age 15, however, the size of the differential varies considerably, both within the United States and among

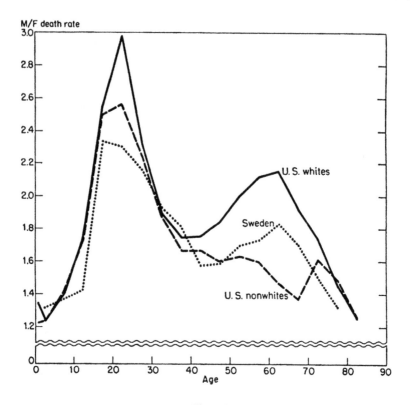

Figure 1
Male–Female Death Rate Ratio, 1967–1968

Sources: U.S. Public Health Service, *Vital Statistics of the United States*, Vol. 2, *Mortality* (Washington, DC: Government Printing Office, 1967, 1968) and U.S. Public Health Service, *Statistical Abstract of Sweden* (Washington, DC: Government Printing Office, 1971).

developed countries. This variation is probably related to an interaction between biological and socioeconomic factors.

As Figure 1 indicates, the male/female mortality ratio in Sweden for young adults is appreciably lower than for U.S. Whites. Again, at ages 45–65 the ratio is considerably lower in Sweden. In both cases the high ratio for U.S. Whites is attributable to relatively high death rates for males, while female rates approach those found in Sweden. As noted previously, among young males the excess deaths in the United States over Sweden are primarily the result of accidents, and in the 45–65 age group the excess is primarily due to heart disease. Although attempts are frequently made to link the lower mortality rates in Sweden to differences in medical care systems, it seems unlikely that these differences are selective for males and females or that they play a significant role in the lower incidence of accidents and heart disease in Swedish men.

Among U.S. Whites the largest sex differentials in mortality are in small southern towns; the smallest are in the suburbs of large northern cities. At young ages, before sex-linked behavioral patterns have had an opportunity to emerge, there are no significant regional differences. For instance, under age 15 the excess of male deaths is 37 percent in the nonmetropolitan counties of the South Atlantic and 36 percent in the metropolitan counties (without central city) of the Middle Atlantic.* At ages 15–64, however, the differentials are 137 percent and 82 percent, respectively. As in the case of the United States–Sweden comparison, it is extremely unlikely that these differences in male/female ratios can be attributed to medical care, income, or the like. The most promising hypothesis is that sex-role differentiation in work and consumption varies sufficiently from one population to another to have significant implications regarding mortality.

The above data are consistent with the view that as female life-styles become more like those of males, differentials in mortality narrow. One study that foreshadows such a trend examined unexpected deaths from heart attacks. In the decade 1949–1959 the ratio of male to female deaths of this type was 12 to 1, but in the period 1967–1971 the ratio was only 4 to 1. In the recent period a majority of the females who died of heart disease were heavy smokers, while only 10 percent had not smoked at all.[11]

MARITAL STATUS

One particularly interesting aspect of sex-related mortality is its relationship to marital status. In all developed countries the unmarried have significantly higher death rates than the married, and this differential is much greater for males than for females: on the average, unmarried males ages 45–54 in developed countries have *double* the death rate of their married counterparts. For females the marital status differential is only 30 percent.

One possible explanation for this is that "life" is produced more efficiently in a husband-wife household and that it is the female who plays the more important role in the process. Thus females who are single, widowed, or divorced can cope

---

*The South Atlantic census division consists of Delaware, Maryland, Virginia, District of Columbia, West Virginia, North Carolina, South Carolina, Georgia, and Florida. The Middle Atlantic division consists of New York, New Jersey, and Pennsylvania.

almost as well as married women, whereas males without spouses seem to be at a much greater disadvantage. One study, moreover, has found a positive effect of the wife's schooling on the husband's health after allowing for many other related variables such as husband's schooling, I.Q., and income.[12]

To be sure, the thread of causality need not run entirely from marital status to health. The marriage market may be selective with respect to health, tending to leave those with poor life expectancy unmarried. This relationship varies considerably from one country to another, however. In the United States about 13 percent of males ages 45–54 are unmarried, and their death rate is 123 percent higher than that of like-aged married males. In the same age group in England and Wales a smaller fraction (11 percent) are unmarried, but their death rate is only 53 percent above the rate for married males. Just as the male-female mortality ratio is higher in the United States than in nearly all other developed countries, so is the unmarried male–married male ratio higher. There is something about life in the United States that is hard on men, particularly on unmarried men. In the United States the probability of death in middle age for an unmarried man is about five times that for a married woman! In England the comparable ratio is only about 2.75.

Among unmarried males in the United States (and in most other developed countries) divorced men have the highest death rate and widowers the next highest, while single men come closest to the married rate. Why should the rates for widowed and divorced men be so much higher than for single men? It could be adverse selection (i.e., the sick and the unstable are the ones who do not remarry). However, the earnings of widowed and divorced men are just as high as the earnings of single men, which tends to refute this hypothesis. Another possible explanation is a decreased desire to live after the loss of a wife. When we examine the mortality ratios of divorced to single males and of widowed to single males by cause of death, we find the highest ratios recorded for suicide, motor accidents, cirrhosis of the liver, homicide, and lung cancer — all causes where a self-destructive behavioral component is very significant. At the other end of the scale, the widowed and divorced rates come closest to the single in the categories of vascular lesions, diabetes, leukemia and aleukemia, and cancer of the digestive organs — all diseases in which identified behavioral decisions play a smaller role.

One does not ordinarily look to poets for insights into health care, but Edna St. Vincent Millay surely expressed a profound truth when she wrote:

> Love cannot fill the thickened lung with breath,
> Nor clear the blood, nor set the fractured bone;
> Yet many a man is making friends with death
> Even as I speak, for lack of love alone.[13]

A Tale of Two States

In the western United States there are two contiguous states that enjoy about the same levels of income and medical care and are alike in many other respects, but their levels of health differ enormously. The inhabitants of Utah are among the healthiest individuals in the United States, while the residents of Nevada are at the opposite end of the spectrum. Comparing death rates of White residents in the two states, for example, we find that infant mortality is about 40 percent higher in Nevada. And lest the reader think that the higher rate in Nevada is attributable to the "sinful" atmosphere of Reno and Las Vegas, we should note that infant mortality in the rest of the state is almost exactly the same as it is in these two cities. Rather, as was argued earlier in this chapter, infant death rates depend critically upon the physical and emotional condition of the mother.

The excess mortality in Nevada drops appreciably for children because, as shall be argued below, differences in life-style account for differences in death rates, and these do not fully emerge until the adult years. As the following figures indicate, the differential for adult men and women is in the range of 40 to 50 percent until old age, at which point the differential naturally decreases.

Excess of Death Rates in Nevada compared
with Utah, Average for 1959–1961 and 1966–1968

AGE GROUP	MALES	FEMALES
<1	42%	35%
1–19	16%	26%
20–39	44%	42%
30–39	37%	42%
40–49	54%	69%
50–59	38%	28%
60–69	26%	17%
70–79	20%	6%

The two states are very much alike with respect to income, schooling, degree of urbanization, climate, and many other variables that are frequently thought to be the cause of variations in mortality. (In fact, average family income is actually higher in Nevada than in Utah.) The numbers of physicians and of hospital beds per capita are also similar in the two states.

What, then, explains these huge differences in death rates? The answer almost surely lies in the different life-styles of the residents of the two states. Utah is inhabited primarily by Mormons, whose influence is strong throughout the state.

Excess of Death Rates in Nevada
compared with Utah for Cirrhosis of the Liver
and Malignant Neoplasms of the Respiratory System,
Average for 1966–1968

AGE	MALES	FEMALES
30–39	590%	443%
40–49	111%	296%
50–59	206%	205%
60–69	117%	227%

Devout Mormons do not use tobacco or alcohol and in general lead stable, quiet lives. Nevada, on the other hand, is a state with high rates of cigarette and alcohol consumption and very high indexes of marital and geographical instability. The contrast with Utah in these respects is extraordinary.

In 1970, 63 percent of Utah's residents 20 years of age and over had been born in the state; in Nevada the comparable figure was only 10 percent; for persons 35–64 the figures were 64 percent in Utah and 8 percent in Nevada. Not only were more than nine out of ten Nevadans of middle age born elsewhere, but more than 60 percent were not even born in the West.

The contrast in stability is also evident in the response to the 1970 census question about changes in residence. In Nevada only 36 percent of persons 5 years of age and over were then living in the same residence as they had been in 1965; in Utah the comparable figure was 54 percent.

The differences in marital status between the two states are also significant in view of the association between marital status and mortality discussed in the previous section. More than 20 percent of Nevada's males ages 35–64 are single, widowed, divorced, or not living with their spouses. Of those who are married with spouse present, more than one-third had been previously widowed or divorced. In Utah the comparable figures are only half as large.

The impact of alcohol and tobacco can be readily seen in the following comparison of death rates from cirrhosis of the liver and malignant neoplasms of the respiratory system. For both sexes the excess of death rates from these causes in Nevada is very large.

The populations of these two states are, to a considerable extent, self-selected extremes from the continuum of life-styles found in the United States. Nevadans, as has been shown, are predominantly recent immigrants from other areas, many of whom were attracted by the state's permissive mores. The inhabitants of Utah, on the other hand, are evidently willing to remain in a more restricted society. Persons born in Utah who do not find these restrictions acceptable tend to move out of the state.

Summary

This dramatic illustration of large health differentials that are unrelated to income or availability of medical care helps to highlight the central themes of this chapter — namely:

1. From the middle of the eighteenth century to the middle of the twentieth century rising real incomes resulted in unprecedented improvements in health in the United States and other developing countries.
2. During most of this period medical care (as distinct from public health measures) played an insignificant role in health, but, beginning in the mid-1930s, major therapeutic discoveries made significant contributions independently of the rise in real income.
3. As a result of the changing nature of health problems, rising income is no longer significantly associated with better health, except in the case of infant mortality (primarily post-neonatal mortality) — and even here the relationship is weaker than it used to be.
4. As a result of the wide diffusion of effective medical care, its marginal contribution to health is again small (over the observed range of variation). There is no reason to believe that the major health problems of the average American would be significantly alleviated by increases in the number of hospitals or physicians. This conclusion might be altered, however, as the result of new scientific discoveries. Alternatively, the *marginal* contribution of medical care might become even smaller as a result of such advances.
5. The greatest current potential for improving the health of the American people is to be found in what they do and don't do to and for themselves. Individual decisions about diet, exercise, and smoking are of critical importance, and collective decisions affecting pollution and other aspects of the environment are also relevant.

These conclusions notwithstanding, the demand for medical care is very great and growing rapidly. As René Dubos has acutely observed, "To ward off disease or recover health, men as a rule find it easier to depend on the healers than to attempt the more difficult task of living wisely."[14]

The next three chapters focus specifically on medical care: physicians, hospitals, and drugs. As discussed in Chapter 1, problems concerning the cost of care and access to care are high on the agenda of the American people. The following chapters provide the background for understanding these problems and for analyzing them from the economic point of view.

Supplementary Reading

Please see "The New Demographic Transition: Most Gains in Life Expectancy Now Realized Late in Life" and "Social Determinants of Health: Caveats and Nuances" in Part 2.

CHAPTER 3

The Physician:
The Captain of the Team

> [The physician's] position in society, the task assigned to him and the rules of conduct imposed upon him changed in every period. They were determined primarily by the social and economic structure of society and by the technical and scientific means available to medicine at the time.
>
> HENRY SIGERIST
> Medicine and Human Welfare

More than 4½ million men and women from some two hundred occupations are employed in the delivery of health services in the United States. One type of health professional — the physician — plays a unique role. Although physicians account for only 8 percent of health service employment, their actions and decisions are of critical importance to the entire system. The term "health team" is sometimes only a figure of speech, but the "captaincy" by the physician is beyond doubt. It is impossible to understand the problems of medical care without understanding the physician. And it is impossible to make significant changes in the medical field without changing physician behavior.

The preeminent position of the physician in medical care is rooted in law, custom, and a more extended training. Historically, the physician *was* the health team. At the beginning of this century, for instance, two out of every three persons employed in the health field were physicians; today the proportion is one out of every twelve. This huge change in the workforce mix is profoundly altering the role of the physician, although medical education and medical practice have all too often failed to adapt to the new circumstances. With the growth of more complex technologies, the changing nature of health problems, and the commitment to serve the total population, a true team effort is required for the successful delivery of health care.

The dominant role of the physician is particularly important with respect to the problem of the *cost* of care. This is not primarily because physicians' fees are too high, though they are in many instances, but because physicians control the total process of care. Typically, this process begins when a patient seeks help. From then on the initiative passes to the physician, whose decisions significantly influence the quantity, type, and cost of service utilized. For instance, the physician, and only the physician, can prescribe drugs. On average, one prescription is written for every outpatient visit; frequently the visit is undertaken primarily to obtain the prescription. The cost of drugs is often as great as the physician's fee, but closer attention by the physician to the choice of drug and brand of drug could significantly reduce that cost.

There are many other decisions that lie solely within the discretion of the physician. One may, for example, order tests or X rays. One may recommend surgery. One may tell the patient to enter the hospital. It is true that the patient is not compelled to follow the physician's advice, but it is equally true that the patient could not obtain the drugs, tests, or hospital admission without the concurrence of the physician. The physician is the gatekeeper to the production of medical care.

The actual delivery of care is frequently in the hands of other health professionals — pharmacists, nurses, technicians, and the like — but they take their instructions from and report back to the physician. For instance, while the pharmacists who fill the prescription are usually independent businesspeople and may even be more knowledgeable about drugs than the physician, they are legally obliged to fill the prescription exactly as written. In many states they cannot so much as substitute one brand of the same drug for another, even though such substitution could result in substantial savings for the patient.

Or consider the role of the physician in the hospital. Typically, physicians are not employees of the institution, but members of the "voluntary" staff and are referred to as "attending" physicians. Although not employees, they have considerable, if not primary, influence over what happens in the hospital. It is they who will decide who enters, what is done to and for the patients while these physicians there, and how long they stay. It is the physicians who, to a large extent, control the activities of such hospital employees as nurses and technicians, who report to them and follow their directions even though they usually occupy no formal position in the hospital chain of command. Not only do physicians influence the day-to-day activities of the hospital, but they play a major role in determining what capital equipment will be purchased and what long-run policies will be followed.

There are, to be sure, changes taking place within the hospital-physician relationship. A significant new development in the United States is the growth of full-time medical staffs. Some hospitals now have senior physicians acting as chiefs of the various services on a salaried basis. There also has been an increase in salaried house staff, particularly interns and residents. These developments modify the role and influence of the "attending" physicians who are not employees of the hospital, but note that the new full-time employees are also physicians. As Dr. Paul Elwood has so well put it, "Hospitals don't have patients; doctors have patients and hospitals have doctors." From the point of view of the hospital administrator, running a hospital is like trying to drive a car when the passengers have control of the wheel and the accelerator. The most the administrator can do is occasionally jam on the brakes.

In many discussions about physicians, primary attention is given to their high fees. "The doctor only saw me for ten minutes and charged $25" is a typical complaint. It is true that physicians' fees have risen more than twice as fast as other consumer prices since the end of World War II and that their incomes have almost doubled in the last decade, but physicians' fees and income are only a small part of the cost problem.

Of every $100 spent for health in the United States only a bit over $20 goes for physicians' services, compared to more than $40 for hospital care and another $10 for drugs. After deducting legitimate expenses for rent, personnel, and supplies, physicians' income represents at most about 15 percent of total health expenditures. This income is admittedly very high, averaging close to $50,000 in 1973. The typical physicians make at least $10,000 more per year than do other highly trained professionals, and their earnings are more than double those of the average college professor.

Part of physicians' high income can be explained by longer and more expensive training and longer hours of work. Most economists believe that part also represents a "monopoly" return to physicians resulting from restrictions on entry to the profession and other barriers to competition. Let us assume that some way could be found to drive down physicians' fees and income to a "competitive" level — that is, to a level commensurate with the training, ability, and effort of the average physician. Such a reduction, even if it cut income by 20 percent while holding utilization constant, would reduce total health costs by only 3 percent.* Clearly the potential saving here is small.

On the other hand, consider the physician's influence on other elements of cost. Expenditures for hospital care and out-of-hospital prescription drugs account for about 50 percent of total health outlays. As we have seen, physician decisions have significant influence on these costs: the volume of surgery, the number of hospital admissions, the length of stay in the hospital, the number and type of prescriptions — all are subject to physician control.

Moreover, there is frequently a wide range of choices open to the physician; it must not be imagined that medical science rigidly determines the appropriate course of treatment. Comparisons within this country and between this country and others reveal wide differences in the use of surgery, drugs, and hospitalization,

---

* Income of physicians (15 percent of total) × 20 percent cut = 3 percent reduction in total.

with significant implications for cost but little apparent effect on health outcomes. For instance, a comparison of surgical procedures performed in an East Coast suburb by physicians practicing under the customary fee-for-service system with the procedures performed by surgeons in a prepaid group practice on the West Coast revealed that 25 percent of the operations for which patients were hospitalized in the East were done on an ambulatory basis in the West, with resulting savings of several hundred dollars per case.[1] No adverse health effects were noted for the nonhospitalized patients; indeed, there may well be more risk when a patient is unnecessarily hospitalized.

Differences in modes of treatment are frequently attributable to institutional differences rather than to differences in the intelligence or competence of the physicians involved. For instance, one of the reasons why more operations are not performed on an ambulatory basis in the East is that sometimes the medical insurance will only pay if the patient is hospitalized, or will pay more for the same procedure if performed on a hospitalized patient.

In the West Coast health plan described above, where patients pay a single annual fee to cover hospitalization, physicians' services, and prescription drugs, the average length of hospital stay for patients with uncomplicated myocardial infarction (heart attack) is ten days compared with a national average of about three weeks. With hospital costs running over $100 per day, the shorter stay represents a saving of over $1,000 per patient for a frequently encountered medical condition. Even more striking are reports from England indicating no difference in health outcomes between heart attack patients who were hospitalized and those who were treated at home.[2]

The elimination of unnecessary surgery, hospital admissions, tests, prescriptions, and the like is the surest, swiftest, safest way of stopping the runaway inflation of health care cost. This goal could be pursued by government regulation or by trying to make the patient more cost-conscious through deductibles and coinsurance. The route that offers the most promise, however, is through informed modification of physician behavior. To accomplish that it is necessary to understand the incentives and constraints that motivate physicians.

A common mistake is to think that the behavior of physicians can be understood only in terms of their desire to maximize income. It is true that physicians' incomes far surpass those of other standard occupations. Most physicians, however, also respond to other kinds of incentives. One significant factor is peer approval. In this respect physicians are very much like writers, artists, athletes, scientists, and performers, all of whom place considerable value on being well regarded by their colleagues. Such high regard can, of course, indirectly yield financial value as well, but it is not unusual for the physician to sacrifice financial reward in order to maintain peer approval. Patient approval is another significant factor that motivates physicians — again, not only because it results in a busier practice and hence more income, but also because of the psychological rewards derived from the dependency relationship frequently established between patient and physician.

Another motivating force in physician behavior is "instinct of workmanship." During their medical school and residency training, physicians are "imprinted" with what they understand to be "best medical practice," to which they try to conform throughout their careers. This can be a mixed blessing because it is closely related to what I have called the "technological imperative" — namely, the desire of the physician to do everything that one has been trained to do, regardless of the benefit-cost ratio.

Other significant influences on physician behavior are the demands of one's family and one's own life-style preferences. The physician's decision regarding where to locate one's practice, for instance, is significantly influenced by the frequent desire to be near cultural, educational, and recreational facilities. Similarly, the preference of most physicians for specialization is partly motivated by a desire to avoid the night calls, house visits, and other demands that disrupt the life of the general practitioner.

Social scientists have tended to criticize the great power that physicians wield in the health care process. Many economists believe that the root of the problem is in licensure laws and other legislation that restrict competition. The case for compulsory licensure (inquiring licenses to practice a profession) presumably rests on the proposition that the consumer is a poor judge of the quality of medical care and therefore needs guidance concerning the qualifications of those proposing to sell such care. Assuming this to be true, *voluntary certification* could provide guidance just as well — indeed, probably better. Under a certification system several grades or categories could be established and periodic recertification required. This would be more practicable — and less threatening — than periodic relicensure because a change in certification would not completely destroy the physicians right to practice. Patients would be free to choose practitioners at whatever level of expertise they wanted, including uncertified practitioners. John Stuart Mill was an early advocate of this position in his famous *Essay on Liberty*. He wrote, "Degrees or other public certificates of scientific or professional acquirements should be given to all who present themselves for examination and stand the test; but such certificates should confer no advantage over competitors other than the weight which may be attached to their testimony by public opinion."

The principal objections to voluntary certification are that some patients might receive bad treatment at the hands of unqualified practitions and that such a system might result in an expansion of unnecessary care. Obvious advantages, on the other hand, are greater availability of care and lower prices. For certain health care needs, practitioners with lesser qualifications than physicians presently have would be adequate — and possibly preferable to a system (like the current one) that results in some sick persons receiving no care or being treated by laypeople without any medical training (such as family members, neighbors, or friends).

A reasonable compromise between the existing restrictive system and complete laissez-faire would be *institutional licensure,* which would restrict care to institutions and organizations that met licensure standards while permitting them considerable freedom and flexibility in the use of personnel. (This approach is discussed in more detail at the end of this chapter.)

Sociologists have been at least as critical of physicians as have economists. Professor Eliott Friedson, for instance, has written, "Health services are organized around professional authority and their basic structure is constituted by the dominance of a single profession over a variety of other subordinate occupations," and goes on to assert that "professional dominance is the analytic key to the present inadequacy of health services."[3] One can sympathize with the thrust of such criticisms, but some nagging questions remain. Why have these laws and customs developed? Why are they present in so many countries with diverse political and economic systems? Are there aspects of the production and delivery of medical care that make these arrangements desirable or, lacking better solutions, the least undesirable one?

Some suggestion of an affirmative answer to the last question can be found in the work of economic theorist Kenneth Arrow. He argues that the *uncertainty* surrounding medical care — that is, uncertainty regarding the need for and the consequences of care — precludes an optimal solution through market competition and gives rise to the various laws and customs that provide the physician with unique power.[4] A related point is that the consumer-provider relationship can significantly affect the effectiveness of medical care. Thus, the arm's-length bargaining position between buyer and seller that is normal and desirable in most markets may actually interfere with the efficient delivery of health services. If I badly need an automobile, I am not likely to reveal to the car dealer the urgency of my demand because it will hurt my chances of a good deal. Furthermore, the utility of the automobile once I purchase it will be unaffected by such bargaining strategy. In medicine, however, lack of candor in giving a history to a physician can significantly reduce the value of the service being purchased. Similarly, the patient's *trust* in the physician often contributes to the cure.

An appreciation of the intimate nature of the relationship between patient and physician and of the desire to be able to fix *responsibility* should make us wary of proposals for radical changes in medical practice. On the other hand, some changes are already taking place, and others should take place.

In evaluating these changes, it is useful to understand the historical forces currently modifying the physician's task. Prior to World War II, the typical American physician was a self-employed general practitioner working alone and delivering a wide variety of services, from maternity to pediatric to geriatric, on a fee-for-service basis. The physician practiced on a small scale presumably because there were no substantial economies to be achieved in large-scale organization. (For similar reasons the traditional practice was also characterized by a low capital-labor ratio.) The physician usually had strong roots in a small town or a well-defined neighborhood of a large city and was substantially involved in the problems of the community. The physician often took a broad view of the doctor's role with respect to health as distinct from medicine, recognized the connections between environment and health, and felt some sense of responsibility for initiating beneficial changes.

This form of practice is not unknown today, but it can no longer be regarded as typical. At present most physicians are specialists in a single branch of medicine, confining their attention to a particular age group, disease, or part of the body. Moreover, fee-for-service practitioners working by themselves are now outnumbered by physicians who practice in groups, who are salaried employees of hospitals, or who otherwise depart from the traditional mode.

These developments are partly in response to changes in medical science. Recent years have seen the development of new diagnostic and therapeutic techniques that require large capital investment and skilled teams of personnel. Improvements in transportation, communication, and information storage and retrieval also have profound implications for the production process in medical care.

Significant changes are also occurring on the side of demand. First, the rapid development of insurance and other types of prepayment has tended to reduce the constraining influence of cost on patients. Second, there has been increasing pressure to distribute medical care more equally regardless of patients' ability to pay. Also, as noted in Chapter 2, there have been major changes in the relative importance of different kinds of health problems. A mode of practice efficiently geared to the detection and treatment of acute infectious diseases may no longer be satisfactory for dealing with the chronic diseases, emotional illness, and other problems that now plague the American people. Finally, it is worth noting that today's physician must deal with a much-better-educated public. At one time physicians were part of an educational elite treating mostly uneducated patients. In 1900 there were five times as many physicians as there were faculty members of colleges and universities. Only in the early 1950s did the number of college teachers catch up with the number of physicians. Now the ratio is more than two to one the other way.

The creation of a health care system that will provide adequate access at reasonable cost requires taking a realistic view of what patients want and need and what physicians actually do. In particular, it requires rejecting the romantic notion that every patient-physician contact is a matter of life or death and recognizing the importance of the *caring* function in medical care.

Caring and Curing

Fully 80 percent of illness is functional, and
can be effectively treated by any talented healer
who displays warmth, interest and compassion
regardless of whether he has finished grammar
school. Another 10 percent of illness is wholly
incurable. That leaves only 10 percent in which
scientific medicine — at considerable cost —
has any value at all.

Letter from a physician to
Medical Economics

One of the central themes of Chapter 2 was that the marginal contribution of
medical care to health in developed countries is very small. While this conclusion
emerged from gross analyses of differences in health across large populations, it
is confirmed by those who have intimate knowledge of medicine and health in
clinical settings. Medical intervention has a significant effect on outcome in only
a small fraction of the cases seen by the average physician. Most illnesses are self-
limiting: they will run their course and disappear. The common cold is a familiar
example. Many others are chronic: given the present limits of medical knowledge,
they are incurable. Arthritis is an all-too-familiar example in this category.

Even this limited capacity of a physician to make a decisive difference is mostly
the result of medical advances of the last fifty years. Prior to that time a patient
had as much chance of being harmed as helped by the treatments of the day.
Describing pre-twentieth-century physicians, Dr. Walsh McDermott writes that
"these rather haphazardly trained and educated men and women provided great
human comfort, but in retrospect it is clear that they had virtually no power to alter
the course of a disease in a predictable and decisive fashion."[5]

Yet the practice of medicine goes back thousands of years, and the demand for
the services of doctors and healers of all types has always been strong. How can
we understand this, if their remedies were so often irrelevant or harmful? This
question is of more than historical interest because the answer may help explain
the current situation as well.

In my view it is critical to appreciate that the physician has always fulfilled a
"caring" as well as a "curing" function. People who are troubled, who are in pain,
who are disabled, want to see someone, to talk to someone, to share their troubles
with someone. As much as a "cure," they want sympathy, reassurance, encouragement. They want explanations: "Why did this happen?" "How long will it last?"
They want justifications: "Should I stay home from work?" "Should I have any
more children?" Above all, they want someone who *cares.*

Doctors, among others, have traditionally fulfilled this function, and it would be a great mistake to believe that it is not still of importance today. Indeed, with the decline of religious belief, the breakup of families, the increase in mobility and anonymity in our urban culture, it may well be that the demand for "caring" is greater than ever before. To quote Dr. McDermott again: "Without question an appreciable portion of what the public voices as the medical services they need and should have, is not really this decisive portion of our medicine at all, but practices that have survived from a day when [physicians] could not act decisively."[6]

Different kinds of physicians encounter the "demand for caring" in different ways. Pediatricians, for instance, know that calming nervous mothers is often more time-consuming than treating their children. Obstetricians must deal with expectant fathers as well as their pregnant spouses. Relieving anxiety is a large part of almost every physician's stock-in-trade. This "noncuring" role of the physician takes many strange forms. In Israel, for example, new immigrants make particularly heavy use of the nationally supported health services. Upon examination it was found that this was not because their medical needs were so much greater than those of the rest of the population, but because using the health service was a means of identifying with this new society, of feeling more a part of the new culture.

"Caring" is particularly important at the close of life, when a "cure" is impossible. Each year some 2 million people die in the United States, in most cases after suffering illness, pain, loss of normal functions, loneliness, and fear. Family, friends, and clergy provide some care, but increasingly this difficult task is being delegated to physicians and other health personnel, especially since more than half of all deaths occur in hospitals or nursing homes.

Although the discussion so far has emphasized the distinction between "caring" and "curing," increasing evidence regarding the connection between psychological states and physical pathology makes it clear that the former can have a significant effect on the latter. In particular, "caring" can be excellent preventive medicine for a patient who has just lost a loved one, say, or suffered some other psychological trauma.

A prominent characteristic of the United States medical care market is that fees are invariably based on the care rendered, not on the cure effected. The almost total divorce of fees and charges from health outcomes makes sense if, as suggested here, it is care that is typically being bought (and sold) and if there is only infrequently a significant relation between care and outcome.

Once we have acknowledged the importance of the "caring" function in the total spectrum of physician activity, several critical questions arise. First, what determines the demand for "caring"? It is obvious that this demand varies greatly among individuals and groups, for levels of anxiety, the need for reassurance about one's health, and the need for sympathy are not constants of human nature. It is also obvious that some part of this demand is satisfied outside the medical care industry in various degrees within different cultures, socioeconomic groups, and "life-styles," although the decline of traditional families and religions in most developed countries has surely expanded the role of health professionals. Still, it is not clear whether such demand arises completely exogenous to medical care or is in part behavior that is learned by patients from physicians.

Another set of questions concerns the ability and willingness of physicians to supply "caring." How well does medical training, which has become increasingly more technical and scientific, prepare physicians for this role? Has the increase in opportunities to help patients by strictly medical means made physicians more intolerant of and dissatisfied with their "caring" function? Should the criteria for admission to medical school take into account the need for this kind of work? One possible solution may be to establish a variety of "hotlines," "drop-in centers," and multiservice organizations managed by volunteers and dedicated para-professionals expert in "caring" by virtue of temperament and/or training. Such a service is probably most effective when provided by someone who "cares" by choice rather than by necessity.

Finally, there are a number of questions that society must face concerning the financing of "caring." How much should this service cost? Who should pay for it? If "caring" is to be provided by physicians with long years of training, it would be very costly — unless the higher price for their time were offset by greater efficiency. What, if any, is the government's obligation in providing "caring," and what are the obligations of individuals and families? When people talk of health care being a "right," or of a "shortage" of care, do they also have "caring" in mind?

Some of these questions will be discussed in Chapter 6, on paying for medical care, and others in the Conclusion. The implications of this subject for the problem of access are considered in the next section.

"I Can't Get a Doctor"

Each physician treateth one part and not more. And everywhere is full of physicians; for some profess themselves physicians of the eyes, and others of the head, others of the teeth, and others of the parts about the belly, and others of obscure sicknesses.

HERODOTUS
(describing Egypt 2,400 years ago)

"I can't get a doctor." So runs the complaint, so often, and in so many places from so many people, one would think that physicians are a vanishing species along with the whooping crane and the California condor. For those who in recent years have experienced great difficulty and delay in securing medical care, it must come as a surprise to learn that the ratio of physicians to population in the United States is higher now than at any time since before World War I. There is actually a higher proportion of physicians in the population of the United States than in Australia, Denmark, England, Japan, the Netherlands, Norway, or Sweden. It may also surprise some to learn that the average annual number of physician-visits per capita, 4.6, is about the same as it was twenty-five years ago and greater than in the pre-World War II period.

Why, then, is *access* perceived as one of the major problems of health care? There are several reasons, some related to changing expectations and demands, and some to the changing nature of medical practice.

First, it should be noted that complaints about access to medical care have their parallel in complaints about the schools, the courts, mass transportation, and so on. Similarly, in affluent suburbs there is an access problem regarding plumbers, electricians, domestic servants, and repair personnel of all types. In short, ours is an age of "great expectations" and little patience — which is not an argument for complacent acceptance of current shortcomings, regarding medical care or anything else, but simply a plea to place these shortcomings into proper perspective.

One contributing factor is the growing ability of the poor to *pay* for care, either in cash, or via private insurance, or through publicly funded programs. A paying patient is likely to apply a different standard than one receiving "free" care. Thus part of the access problem is related to the fact that care is being distributed more equally than ever before; among groups (particularly the poor) who now have better access than formerly there are those who tend to forget how bad things once were or are simply unaware of the enormous problems their parents faced. Moreover, even though access for them may be better, it may still leave much to be desired. On the other hand, among groups (particularly the wealthy) who have suffered a deterioration in access there are those who remember all too well when physicians would come running at the call of a promptly paying patient.

Probably the most important reason for current complaints about access, however, is the growth of specialty practice within medicine, which has made it more difficult to gain access to primary care, access to emergency care, access to the medical system itself. A related phenomenon is the change in control of the *terms* of access. In earlier times a patient could decide pretty much when and where the doctor visit would take place: frequently this was at home, and just as often as not it would be at night or on a weekend. Today's specialist sees the patients only at certain specified hours, usually in one's office or in the hospital.

The growth of specialization has also contributed to the phenomenon of patients making greater distinctions among physicians. Mr. Jones complains that he has to wait six weeks to be operated on by Dr. X, and doesn't bother to mention that

Drs. Y or Z, who have passed their boards in the same specialty, would be happy to take the case tomorrow. (See the next section on the "surgeon surplus.")

Another difficulty often cited is in finding a physician who will take continuing responsibility for the whole patient. A generation ago more than half of all active physicians were general practitioners; now only one out of seven is in general practice. Specialists in internal medicine have tended to fill the need for "first-contact" general care, but many younger internists prefer to limit their practice to a subspecialty, such as cardiology, hematology, or endocrinology.

What the typical patient wants is easy, quick, reliable access to a source of care seven days a week, twenty-four hours a day. Moreover, patients want this source to know them, have all their records, care about them, take continuing responsibility for them, and guide them through the labyrinth of whatever specialty care may be necessary. Such access is indeed rare. Instead, the medical care industry offers patients a multitude of highly trained specialists, each of whom can provide better care than was previously available — but only within one's specialty and only during office hours.

In my view the patient's demand for access cannot be met for the total population by personnel now known as physicians — that is, highly skilled specialists with ten to twelve years of training beyond high school. Such personnel are not only too expensive, but also frequently illsuited to meet the typical demands of most first-contact situations.

An efficient, effective solution to the access problem requires the deployment of properly trained, properly supervised nurse clinicians, physician's assistants, pediatric assistants, family health workers, and other health professionals. The exact form of organization can vary. One far-seeing physician, Dr. Sidney Garfield, one of the pioneers of the Kaiser Health Plan, advocates the organization of care around four centers of activity: (1) A triage (screening) center for the worried well; (2) a health-maintenance center for immunization and other care of the well; (3) a center for the chronically ill; and (4) an acute care center. Only in the last would the bulk of patient contact be with physicians. In the others, physicians would help to design and monitor diagnostic and therapeutic protocols and would be available for consultation, but most of the patient contact would be with other health professionals.[7] One reason why it is currently so difficult to get care in time of need is because physicians' offices and hospitals are full of people who are not acutely ill. The four-tiered organization of health services would thus facilitate access for all — those who are acutely ill as well as those who are not.

No discussion of the problem of access would be complete without reference to geographic disparities in the availability of physicians. It is perfectly clear that physicians prefer to locate in urban areas. The number of physicians per capita is three times as high in metropolitan counties as in nonmetropolitan counties in the United States. The average physician in nonmetropolitan counties sees about one-third more patients per week, but that still leaves a disparity of more than two to one. The relative shortage of physicians in rural areas is not peculiar to the United States; it is true of almost every country. It is not a function of the national physician/population ratio, or of the method of financing health care, or of the type of economy. The basic reason for geographic inequality is the same in every country: the reluctance of physicians to live and practice in remote areas. Of course, medical care is not the only service that is relatively scarcer in rural areas. Cultural, educational, and recreational facilities are usually scarce as well — which, as we have already mentioned, is a principal reason why physicians prefer urban locations.

Comparisons of the health levels of inhabitants of rural and urban areas do not suggest that the former are significantly worse off on balance. Living in low-density areas undoubtedly has offsetting advantages: fresh air, beautiful scenery, privacy. Rural death rates tend to be slightly higher than urban rates for infants, children, and young adults, but after age 45 the differential is in favor of rural areas. Thus if American country dwellers suffer from their lower physician/population ratio, it is primarily in terms of convenience, not of health.

Geographical inequality is often cited as a reason for increasing the total number of physicians in the country. Presumably, the resultant excess in the number of physicians in certain areas would induce some to move to areas with lower physician/population ratios. But if we test this theory by examining the four regions of the United States (Northeast, North Central, South, and West) and comparing each region's overall physician/population ratio with the degree of internal geographic inequality, the argument is dramatically refuted. The two regions with the highest physician/population ratios — the Northeast and the West — also exhibit the greatest relative inequality among their states. Within the North Central region and the South, with much lower physician/population ratios, there is much *less* intraregional inequality.

Certainly this is not to suggest that an increase in the total number of physicians in the United States would not result in some absolute increase in rural areas as well. But there is no reason to believe that if the total supply were much larger than now, the *relative* disparity between urban and rural areas would be any less. Moreover, increasing the number of physicians as they are now being trained would involve a significant waste of resources, for some specialties, such as surgery, are already in oversupply.

The "Surgeon Surplus"

The "doctor shortage" has become a stock phrase in almost every speech and article about American medical care. As suggested in the preceding section, this is an accurate characterization for some types of care. For some medical services, particularly house calls and emergency care, the quantity demanded at the going price is greater than the quantity supplied. But there are other kinds of medical services where the opposite situation prevails. For most types of surgery, the quantity physicians would like to supply at the going price is far greater than the quantity demanded. In the opinion of most experts, within both medicine and economics, there is indeed a "surgeon surplus."

The existence and extent of this surplus have been discussed from a number of different points of view. At the clinical level, experienced surgeons have known for a long time that there is not enough "business" to keep everyone as active as they would like to be. Back in 1965 Dr. William P. Longmire wrote, "In each community in our country there are a few surgeons who are doing all or more than they humanly can do. Many, though, are working at a pace far below their capacity and this is a tremendous waste of highly skilled talent."[8] In his inaugural address as president of the American College of Surgeons in 1972, Dr. Longmire went so far as to propose limiting the number of surgical training residencies in order to bring about a better balance between supply and demand.

Professor John Bunker, a leading anesthesiologist, in 1970 compared the situations in the United States and England and found that there were twice as many surgeons per capita in this country and twice as much surgery being performed here. Some procedures, particularly those for which indications are frequently in doubt (such as tonsillectomy), were found to be three or four times as prevalent here.

A comprehensive, detailed study of general surgeons in one suburban community in the New York metropolitan area revealed that the surgical workload of the typical surgeon was only about *one-third* of what experts deemed a reasonably full schedule. Furthermore, the uneven distribution of work was quite marked. The busiest person in the community was very busy, doing more than four times as much surgery as the average surgeon. One-fourth of the surgeons were doing 50 percent of the surgery; their average work load was triple that of their colleagues.

This study also revealed that a large part of the surgical work load in the community consisted of relatively simple procedures. For instance, more than half the operations were less complex than a simple herniorrhaphy. The repair of hernia, which is one of the most common general surgical procedures, is a task which is often assigned to surgical residents in their first year of training.[9]

There is no reason to believe that the findings from this study are atypical of the general situation. Calculations based on the total number of surgeons and the total volume of operations in New York State revealed about the same average work loads, and similar calculations for the United States produced results that were only slightly higher.

By, contrast, in organized health care settings where the number of surgeons employed is geared to patient requirements, the average work load is much higher. In one prepaid group practice the average surgeon was found to be performing more than twice as much surgery as those in the suburban private practice setting previously discussed. Moreover, the work load was very evenly distributed among all the surgeons in the groups. A large fee-for-service multispeciality clinic in which all physicians are on salary reports an even higher average work load — more than three times the national average. In this clinic extensive use of assistants in the operating room helps to maintain the high level of productivity. The most important factor accounting for surgical productivity in any setting, however, is limiting the number of surgeons relative to the work to be done.

One might think that a surgeon without enough surgery to do would spend more time in other kinds of medical work, such as general practice. With the surgeons in the New York suburb mentioned above, however, this was not the case; rather they were enjoying a great deal of leisure. On the job they appeared to be very busy, but when account was taken of long weekends, days off, afternoons off, and the like, it was found that they were at work only an average of thirty-four hours per week.[10] This was based on a generous definition of "at work" to include all the hours from the time a surgeon first appeared at hospital or office until one went home. Thus time for lunch and personal business were included in "at work."

Do surgeons with such small work loads find it difficult to make a living? In this case not at all, for fee levels were high enough to insure that even those with small practices made a comfortable living, and the surgeons with the heaviest work loads had very high incomes because the level of fees was generally about the same for all surgeons in the community. If fees were set as they are in the Netherlands — by establishing a reasonable income level and a reasonable work load for surgeons and then dividing the former figure by the latter — the result would be a sharp reduction in cost to the consumer. For instance, suppose a gross income of $60,000 per year from in-hospital surgery were considered appropriate for a general surgeon. (This surgeon's total gross would include income from the office practice.) The equivalent of four hundred herniorrhaphies, requiring about ten hours per week in the operating room, is a reasonable annual work load. Therefore, under the system described above the fee for a herniorraphy would be $150, which is less than half the fee now charged in most major American markets.

Why doesn't competition among all these surgeons drive down fees and eventually force some to turn to other kinds of work? The answer to this is not clear, although one reason seems to be that lowering fees might provoke one's colleagues to deny a surgeon hospital privileges or seek to damage one's reputation. Also, many surgeons believe, perhaps rightly, that demand would not increase appreciably in response to a price cut, so they might wind up making less rather than more money. There is one kind of price cutting that this situation does encourage, however, and that is fee splitting. In this practice, which is considered unethical, the surgeon kicks back part of the patient's fee to the physician who referred the patient for surgery. Even in the absence of fee splitting, surgeons usually make strenuous efforts to cultivate the goodwill of internists, general practitioners, and other physicians who are in a position to refer patients.

The existence of a "surgeon surplus" is fairly common knowledge within the profession. Why then are so many new surgeons being turned out every year? (Between 1950 and 1970, for example, the number of surgical residencies offered in the United States increased by over 100 percent!) One reason is that those responsible for the creation of new surgical residencies are not the same people who have to contend with excess supply after training has been completed.

The push for residencies comes from the surgical chiefs in hospitals, who are frequently full-time salaried physicians not involved in private practice and who like having a great many young physicians receiving training under them because it enhances their own position and provides them with abundant assistance in their clinical and research tasks. In addition, at least until recently, hospital administrators wanted a great many residents around because they were useful in providing medical care in the emergency room, on the wards, and the like. In other words, residents were a cheap source of skilled labor.

Because hospitals frequently use residents for duties only distantly related to their training needs, and because the supply of surgeons tends to exceed the demand for surgery, many surgical residency programs can only provide the resident with sufficient operating experience by prolonging the training period. Thus the training program is often drawn out to five or even six years, partly because there is not enough clinical "material" to go around.[11] A recent study of a surgeon-training program in a supposedly busy municipal hospital in New York City revealed that the surgical residents were actually doing very little surgery until their fifth year of training because of a shortage of cases requiring surgery.[12]

According to some critics, the existence of "excess capacity" among surgeons results in considerable "unnecessary" surgery. This is a highly controversial point, since it is frequently difficult to state with absolute certainty whether any operation is justified or not. It does seem to be true that physicians practicing in prepaid health plans are less likely to recommend surgery than those practicing fee-for-service. It also has been reported that making a second medical opinion mandatory before proceeding with surgery tends to reduce the number of operations.[13]

Defenders of traditional medical practice assert that only a small fraction of surgeons are "greedy" and likely to perform unnecessary surgery. This may well be true — but, the surgical work loads of these surgeons may be larger than average, and thus the proportion of unnecessary operations might be higher than the proportion of greedy surgeons. And since the average patient comes under the care of many different surgeons during one's lifetime, the chances of undergoing an unnecessary operation may not be small even if the fraction of surgeons who are greedy is small.

In fairness to physicians it should be noted that some unnecessary surgery is probably the result of patient pressure rather than surgical greed. Parents of children with recurrent sore throats and similar problems frequently insist on tonsillectomies, and the high volume of hysterectomies among American women may say something about the women as well as their physicians.

Also in fairness to surgeons it should not be thought that every procedure and service ordered by internists and other physicians is of unquestionable value. There are vast numbers of cases where opinions concerning the proper course of treatment differ substantially, and the charge of "unnecessary" could be leveled against certain tests, X rays, visits, and injections with as much justification as against certain operations.

Even if it led to no unnecessary surgery at all, however, the surgeon surplus would still pose problems: it raises the overall cost of medical care, it prolongs the period of training, and it results in some surgeons losing valuable skills because they operate so infrequently. From both the economic and health points of view, a more rational approach to training and utilizing the surgical workforce — and medical specialists in general — is badly needed.

Meeting the Challenge

The challenge facing American medicine is to devise a system of medical care that provides ready access at reasonable cost. In my view such a system would make extensive use of "physician extenders" practicing within licensed institutions. These physician extenders — variously known as physicians' assistants, nurse clinicians, pediatric assistants, nurse practitioners, and the like — would have considerably shorter training than physicians and would function in organized settings under physicians' guidance and supervision, performing many of the tasks now reserved by law and tradition for physicians. It has been repeatedly shown that today's physician, with intensive training in specialty and subspecialty care, is too expensive and sometimes poorly suited to provide the primary, preventive, and emergency care which lie at the heart of the present access problem. Thus the availability of large numbers of physician extenders offers the promise of simultaneously lowering the cost of care, improving access, and possibly even raising health levels.

Some physician extenders are already at work in a variety of settings. Controlled studies of the care they deliver compared with conventional care by physicians have shown no diminution in quality and frequently enhanced patient satisfaction. In pediatric care, for instance, nurse practitioners were found to be more thorough in their examinations and in their communication with mothers than pediatricians who are frequently bored with the routine aspects of well-baby care. In a study of services for chronically ill patients, nurse practitioners working in consultation with physicians achieved health outcomes and patient satisfaction at least as high as when physicians had complete responsibility. Many physician extenders can relate more closely to patients and their problems, communicate better with them, and afford to spend more time with individual patients.

The number of training programs for physician extenders has grown at an extremely rapid rate. It is now possible to note several different types that will be coming into the health field. Some who are generalists are expected to work in rural settings with considerable independence except for consultation with physicians. Others will work more closely with primary-care physicians as assistants and assume less independent responsibility. Still others will receive specialized training and work with specialized physicians, such as orthopedic surgeons or urologists.

Numerous questions inevitably arise concerning the licensing of such personnel and their compensation. In the opinion of many experts it is of critical importance that the government avoid creating another spectrum of licensed health professionals practicing in a solo, fee-for-service mode. The power to issue licenses rests with individual states, some of which now license as many as two dozen separate health occupations. Such licensure ostensibly protects the public interest, but an increasing number of observers have begun to question whether it in fact serves that purpose.

A license to practice a health profession is usually granted early in a person's career; renewal is practically automatic regardless of subsequent changes in competence. Revocation or suspension of one's license is extremely rare; the percentage so affected is much smaller than the probable incidence of drug addiction, alcoholism, criminal behavior, or insanity in the numbers licensed.

According to the 1973 report of the Federal Commission on Medical Malpractice, only fifteen states permit a physician's license to be challenged on the ground of professional incompetence, and most state medical practice acts have no adequate provision for disciplining those practitioners who are in fact found to be incompetent.[14]

Because holding an individual license is now essential to practice, regulatory agencies and courts are extremely loath to revoke a physician's license, even when there are strong grounds for doing so. In one California case a physician was charged with gross incompetence in 1966, but the final court order suspending his license for ninety days and thereafter restricting his privileges was not issued until 1972. Other physicians have been allowed to continue to practice even after having been found guilty of fraud or comparable criminal acts.

The requirement of licensure often prevents persons who may be well qualified from providing needed services because they lack the degrees or other formal requirements for a license. Work experience and on-the-job training, which often help ambitious, able men and women move up the occupational ladder in other industries, does not facilitate upward mobility in the health field.

One suggested remedy is the substitution of institutional licensure for the licensing of individuals. Under such a system medical care institutions — hospitals, clinics, physicians' groups, etc. — would be licensed by the state and would then be free to hire and use personnel as each saw fit. As two leading advocates of institutional licensing have written:

> The state institutional licensing agency would require that the health institution use only objective criteria relating to the safe and competent performance in the particular position.... The list of legally relevant factors [that institutions would consider in hiring and utilizing personnel] would no longer be limited to the status of being licensed, which is often of little or no value in assigning employees to particular positions, but would include criteria of formal education, job experience, in-service training and other relevant factors.[15]

This approach offers numerous advantages to both consumers and providers. It would permit a much more efficient deployment of health care personnel as well as provide greater opportunity for upward job mobility. And it would no doubt foster the development of a more rational health workforce mix. In most industries there is a continuum of personnel with respect to skills and earnings, with the heaviest concentration in the middle ranges. The health care field, by contrast, is characterized by a bimodal distribution in which very few persons' incomes fall between the arithmetic mean and twice the mean (see Figure 1).[16]

Institutional licensure would also help simplify and rationalize the state's control of medical care. At present there are within each state many health licensing

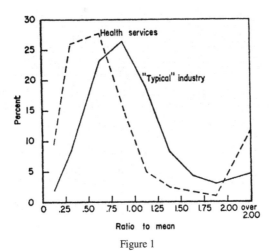

Figure 1

Percentage Frequency Distributions of Earnings Relative to the Mean, Health Services, and the "Typical" Industry, 1959

Sources: Victor R. Fuchs, Elizabeth Rand, and Bonnie Garrett, "The Distribution of Earnings in Health and Other Industries," *Journal of Human Resources* 5, no. 3 (Summer 1970).

agencies (usually one per occupation), and many are dominated by representatives of the occupations they are supposed to control. Institutional licensure would require but a single state medical licensing agency that could and should be dominated by public representatives.

What would be the fate of the physician under such a system? Would one still be "captain of the team"? Certainly in most cases one would be, by virtue of one's more advanced training and knowledge. Indeed, the demands on the physician to play a true leadership role would be greater than they are under the present system of fragmented care. Some physicians would undoubtedly continue to function as highly specialized technicians in particular aspects of medicine or surgery. Many others, however, would not be directly or continuously involved in the personal delivery of care to patients, but would instead assume overall responsibility for the health of the population served. In such a role they would have to be a source of leadership, guidance, inspiration, and control for the entire health care team. Someone other than a physician might conceivably take this leadership role, although the need for expert knowledge and for someone whose authority is readily accepted by patients and health professionals alike make physicians the logical choice in most instances.

Would physicians accept such a role? Some might resist for fear of suffering reduction in income. But as was pointed out earlier in this chapter, the principal economic savings are to be achieved by changing the way physicians practice, not by reducing their compensation. Besides representing to physicians a financial threat, real or imagined, the changes suggested here imply modifying the physician's role. This shift is the inevitable result of technological, economic, political, and social forces which should not be blindly resisted. Physicians, Henry Sigerist noted, "look back to a task that has gone irrevocably; trained as highly specialized and efficient scientists, they are unprepared to grapple with problems that are primarily social and economic. They have built for themselves a legendary, sentimental and romantic history of their profession to which they cling desperately, and which determines their actions."[17]

Many of the present generation of physicians, trained for a more traditional practice, will undoubtedly view the changes recommended here as tending to diminish the compassion and humanity that they associate with the practice of medicine. The next generation, however, trained in new ways for new responsibilities, may prove to be more compassionate, more humane, and more devoted than the old.

Supplementary Reading

Please see "The Structure of Medical Education — It's Time For a Change" and "The Doctor's Dilemma — What is Appropriate Care?" in Part 2.

CHAPTER 4

The Hospital:
The House of Hope

The hospital has evolved from a House of
Despair avoided by all but the impoverished
sick to a House of Hope to which all roads
lead in time of crisis — be it somatic, psychic
or social in origin.

JOHN H. KNOWLES, M.D.
"The Medical Center and the
Community Health Center," in
Social Policy for Health Care

The American hospital is large, impersonal, and dominated by elaborate technology. The American hospital is small, inefficient, underequipped, and understaffed. The American hospital exists primarily to further the professional and economic interests of physicians. The American hospital exists to serve the community. The American hospital is crowded to the point of inefficiency and even danger, and serious delays are encountered in obtaining admission. The American hospital is often half-empty, and many of its patients should be at home or in extended-care facilities. The American hospital is the noblest expression of the philanthropic impulse. The American hospital is a business run to show a profit for its owners.

Will the "real" American hospital please stand up? Which of these many contradictory characterizations of United States hospitals is correct? To some extent, all of them are. No other country has such a heterogeneous collection of institutions comprising its hospital "system." In no other country is it as difficult to generalize about hospitals or to analyze their strengths and shortcomings. If it is important to recognize that American hospitals come in all shapes and sizes, it is equally important to realize that they are undergoing substantial change. This chapter is intended to provide both a still portrait of hospitals as they exist today and a motion picture of the changes that are under way.

The original function of hospitals was to provide the poor with a place to die. The ability of these hospitals to improve health outcomes was sharply limited by the paucity of medical knowledge, as discussed in Chapter 2. Until this century, wealthy individuals who were sick could usually find more comfort, cleanliness, and service in their own homes than in hospitals.

With the development of modern medicine the function of the hospital changed, and it became "the doctor's workshop." The image of the hospital changed from being a place to die to the place where good, effective medical cures could be obtained. Today numerous illnesses can be much more effectively diagnosed and treated in the hospital; for some procedures, such as major surgery, hospitalization is essential.

Now another change is in process. Some hospitals are beginning to function as "health care centers" for the community. The changing nature of health problems and of medical practice, the changing relationship between physicians and hospitals, and the explosive growth in numbers of health personnel other than physicians are all factors in this reorientation. According to many observers, hospitals should now be putting more emphasis on preventive medicine, health education, ambulatory care, home care, rehabilitation services, and responsibility for patients in other institutions (such as extended-care facilities). For the most part these are still matters for discussion rather than actual implementation, but they point to significant changes that lie ahead.

The Central Problem — High Cost

While many kinds of criticisms have been levied against American hospitals, the central problem at present is the high and rapidly rising *cost* of care. In 1973 the operating expenditures of U.S. hospitals plus the cost of new hospital construction amounted to approximately $40 billion, representing more than 40 percent of that year's total national health expenditures. In other words, Americans were spending almost $200 per person for this one aspect of medical care. Not only are costs high, but they have been rising at an extremely rapid rate — more than 10 percent annually over the past decade. It is the escalation in hospital costs that is threatening to blow our medical care system sky high; it is hospital costs that must be curbed if we are ever to bring the system under control.

The high cost of hospital care is attributable in large part to overutilization, inefficiency, and excess capacity resulting from the way current operations and capital investment are financed. Only a small fraction of the cost of hospital care is paid for directly by patients; the bulk comes from so-called third parties, of which the government is the most important, picking up over half the total bill. Private insurance pays about one-third, and the balance is accounted for by private philanthropy. Until recently, the third-party payers made very little effort to question the size of hospital bills. Matters such as weighing the necessity of admission and determining the appropriate length of stay were, and to a large extent still are, left to the professional judgment of the physician and are not to be questioned by "financial intermediaries." The rate of reimbursement for each hospital is determined primarily by *its* costs. Thus, high-cost hospitals are rewarded with higher reimbursement. Capital for construction of new hospitals or expansion of old ones comes primarily from government or philanthropy and does not necessarily flow to communities or institutions that demonstrate efficiency in providing for effective demand. This system is changing, but very slowly.

The deficiencies of the traditional financing system are compounded by the fact that most key decisions are made by physicians who typically have no financial stake in keeping down hospital costs. Indeed, their own self-interest is frequently served by decisions which raise the cost of care. As J. Douglas Colman, the late head of New York's Blue Cross, maintained:

> We must remember that most elements of hospital and medical care costs are generated or based on professional medical judgement. The judgements include the decision to order various diagnostic or therapeutic procedures for patients, and the larger decision as to the types of facilities and services needed by an institution for proper patient care. For the most part, these professional judgements are rendered outside of any organizational structure that fixes accountability for the economic consequences of these judgements.[1]

Before taking a more detailed look at the cost problem and what can be done about it, a brief overview of the economics of the hospital industry will be useful.

Hospitals Today

In the United States there are just over seven thousand hospitals containing more than 1½ million beds. They employ more than 2½ million persons, admit more than 33 million patients annually for inpatient care, and provide over 200 million outpatient visits per year. Hospitals differ in many ways: by type of ownership, type of patient, number of beds, and so on. Probably the most important distinction is between the so-called short-term community hospitals and all others. Community hospitals have only a little over one-half of all hospital beds, but they account for 92 percent of all admissions and 78 percent of all hospital expenses. The "all others" category includes hospitals operated by the federal government, such as Veterans Administration hospitals; psychiatric hospitals, typically operated by states or counties; tuberculosis hospitals (rapidly disappearing); and other hospitals for long-term care.

The most distinctive feature of the community hospital is short average length of stay — the typical patient stays for less than eight days. In psychiatric hospitals, by contrast, the average length of stay is about eight months, and even this represents a considerable shortening from twenty years ago, when the average was about two years.

Because most admissions, personnel, and expenses are concentrated in community hospitals, they have received the most attention from researchers and policy makers. The discussion below follows that precedent, with particular emphasis on differences in the size, ownership, and location of community hospitals.

HOSPITAL SIZE

Hospital size is typically measured in terms of number of beds, and efficiency in terms of expenditures per case or expenditures per patient-day. It is difficult to make precise determinations of the effect of size on efficiency because hospitals that differ in size frequently differ also with respect to location, kind of patient admitted, services provided, extent of teaching responsibilities, and other characteristics that affect expenditures. As the result of a number of studies that have attempted to take account of these variables, however, a broad consensus is emerging. According to most health economists, substantial economies of scale (increasing efficiency) are associated with larger hospital size, at least until about 200 beds; some investigators believe that further gains are possible up to about 500 beds. A few prefer hospitals as large as 1,000 beds, although there are others who argue that this size is too big to be truly efficient.

One of the most interesting studies of the effect of size on costs, by John Carr and Paul Feldstein, found that this relationship varied with the number of services and facilities offered by the hospital. The authors concluded that "small hospitals with high service capability should not generally be built because they are likely to be of uneconomic size. Large hospitals having low service capability are also likely to be uneconomic, since there are few or no additional economies associated with increased size."[2] In other words, if hospitals are not going to provide a large number of complex services, they needn't be very large to be efficient; but if they are to provide a large number of services, it is very inefficient for them to be small. A hospital of 200 beds can efficiently provide most of the basic services needed for routine short-term care — radiology, laboratory, nursing, and the like. Should that hospital grow to 600 beds and still provide only the same basic services, some inefficiencies are likely to develop because of increasing difficulties of administrative control. What is likely to happen, however, is that more specialized services will emerge in the 600-bed unit, services which couldn't possibly have been provided at a reasonable cost when the hospital had only 200 beds.

Persons with direct experience in running hospitals tend to confirm the results of such econometric studies. The president of one major corporation that owns and operates a large chain of for-profit hospitals personally told me that his company would rather not build or operate one that had fewer than 200 beds, but they would be equally apprehensive about a hospital with more than 500 beds.

Given these views about hospital size, it is of interest and concern to note that many American hospitals are too small and some are probably too large. Despite the reservations of many experts about the ability of small hospitals to deliver efficient, high-quality care, *most* "community" (nonfederal, short-term general) hospitals have fewer than 200 beds. In fact, almost 40 percent of the hospital *beds* in the United States are in such "small" hospitals. Another 40 percent of the beds are in "medium-size" hospitals (those with from 200 to 500 beds), and 20 percent are in "large" hospitals (over 500 beds).

Statistics published by the American Hospital Association reveal some important differences among hospitals of different size, especially between small hospitals and those with over 200 beds.* For instance, occupancy rates average only about 70 percent of capacity in small hospitals, while they are over 80 percent in the medium-size and large hospitals. Some excess capacity in the hospital system is desirable in order to meet peak and emergency demands, but an average occupancy rate of 70 percent is too low.†

The relationship among occupancy rate, size of hospital, and size of community served is a complex one. In theory, the size of the community should be the major influence. A small community needs relatively more excess capacity in order to provide the same degree of protection against random fluctuations in the demand for hospital care. Many small hospitals in fact serve communities with small populations, but many do not. In fact, well over one thousand small hospitals are located in metropolitan areas, where low occupancy rates represent a significant waste because the excess capacity cannot be justified in terms of community needs. Furthermore, improvements in transportation and communication diminish the need for small hospitals even in some areas of low population density.

Judging by average length of stay, the more seriously ill tend to get treated in the larger hospitals: the 1971 average-stay figures were 7.2 days for small hospitals, 8.1 days for medium-size hospitals, and 9.8 days for large ones. Some of the difference in average stay, however, may be due to the presence of teaching programs in larger hospitals or to inefficiencies that develop in large, complex institutions. Curiously, the small hospitals do not account for a disproportionate number of maternity cases, one of the simpler types of hospital admissions. In 1971, one out of ten admissions in small hospitals was for childbirth; in the others the ratio was one out of eight.

The number of hospital personnel per patient varies directly with hospital size. The 1971 ratios were 2.7, 3.0, and 3.4, respectively. Such differences are probably attributable to the tendency for larger hospitals to have sicker patients and more research and teaching responsibilities. Only 3 percent of the small hospitals have residency programs, compared with half of the medium-size ones and 90 percent of the large hospitals.

---

*The statistics used in the following discussion are from *Hospitals: Journal of the American Hospital Association,* Guide Issue, Part 2 (1972).

†Hospital administrators consider the optimum occupancy rate to be about 85 percent.

One of the most striking differences among hospitals is in the amount of capital investment. Assets per bed for hospitals with over 200 beds are about 40 percent greater than in the small hospitals. The relationship with size is much weaker among larger hospitals; the asset/bed ratio for those with over 500 beds is only 4 percent greater than those in the 200–500-bed category.

Differences in capital investment are reflected clearly in the data on availability of facilities and services by size of hospital. For instance, nearly all hospitals with over 200 beds have postoperative recovery rooms, but one-third of the small hospitals do not. And two-thirds of the small hospitals don't have intensive-care units. The percentages in small hospitals of other facilities and services that tend to be standard in medium-size and large hospitals are as follows: full-time registered pharmacist, 43 percent; diagnostic radioisotopic facility, 22 percent; histopathology lab, 29 percent; blood bank, 53 percent; inhalation therapy, 48 percent; and physical therapy department, 53 percent.

Of some forty-two facilities and services listed by the American Hospital Association, the mean percentage available in small hospitals is 19 percent. In hospitals in the 200–500-bed range the mean is 46 percent, and in those with over 500 beds it is 64 percent. Facilities and services that are much more frequently available in large than in medium-size hospitals are open-heart surgery, cobalt therapy, renal dialysis, occupational therapy, and numerous psychiatric services.

It is certainly not my intention in this discussion to suggest that these expensive facilities should be available in more hospitals. Indeed, there is considerable evidence that some of them, such as open-heart-surgery units, have proliferated far beyond the limits dictated by medical need or financial prudence.[3] A facility that is seldom used is not only wasteful of resources, but cannot deliver the same quality of care as one that is in regular use. The above statistics nevertheless serve to highlight the fact that hospitals differ greatly in the range of services they can provide. What is desperately needed is some sort of *systematic* approach to meeting the hospital care needs of a region, avoiding unnecessary duplication and insuring that patients are appropriately placed to receive the necessary services. There are probably some services that no hospital should be without, and institutions that are too small to provide them efficiently ought to be phased out of operation. Beyond that, all the hospitals in a given area should be functionally integrated so that there can be an easy flow of patients and physicians from one facility to another depending upon medical requirements and available space.

No one should imagine that such a rational system is easily put into effect. As indicated in Chapter 3, the typical hospital is dominated by the physicians who practice in it. A physician who has the privilege (that is the word used) of admitting patients to a hospital has a competitive advantage over physicians who have no such privilege. The admitting privilege may be obtained by having gone through a prestigious medical school and postgraduate training program, through family or other personal connections, by demonstrations of skill, by agreeing to provide free time for teaching or the care of charity patients, and in other ways. The practice of limiting admitting privileges to certain physicians is commonly defended as a necessary means of controlling the quality of care in the institution. This is probably a valid claim, but the system also limits competition and contributes to the fragmentation of the hospital system. It can also contribute to unnecessary utilization to the extent that physicians can be pressured to fill beds under pain of losing their admitting privileges when demand for hospital care is low.

Hospital trustees are also often a source of difficulty. Many hold their positions because of past or prospective financial contributions, and they are emotionally attached to "their" hospitals. At present philanthropy accounts for only a very small part of total hospital expenditures, but the philanthropists or their descendents continue to have a disproportionate degree of influence in hospital affairs. The notion of merging with a better-managed hospital, or of going out of business altogether, is not easily accepted by those with a large emotional stake in a particular hospital.

Institutional change is never easy, for any industry. The present system of hospital financing does not provide physicians or hospital trustees with enough incentives to undertake socially desirable reorganizations, nor does it impose punishments for failure to do so.

TYPE OF OWNERSHIP

Community hospitals are typically private nonprofit organizations. Many were founded by religious groups; others were established as a result of community-wide efforts or the benefactions of a few secular philanthropists. About one-fourth of the beds are in hospitals owned and operated by state or local governments, and 6 percent are in "proprietary" hospitals, that is, hospitals privately owned and run for profit.

The influence of type of ownership on the effectiveness, efficiency, and equity of care provided has always been a matter of considerable debate. Most people in the health field are strongly opposed to hospitals run for profit, primarily on the grounds that it is "wrong to make a profit out of illness," while ignoring the fact that this is precisely what physicians, pharmacists, and others do. Specific criticisms of for-profit hospitals are that they do not provide care for those who cannot pay, that they do not engage in teaching or research, and that they selectively admit the less seriously ill, thus "skimming the market." Certainly not every hospital need be engaged in teaching and research, however, nor is there any good reason for every hospital to have the personnel and facilities to deliver tertiary care* to very sick patients with complicated conditions.

---

*Care rendered by specialists to patients who have been referred by other physicians, usually for complicated and serious health problems.

As economists have begun paying more attention to the hospital field, the private nonprofit institutions have come in for substantial criticism. They are, it is asserted, inefficient and lacking in adequate incentives; they carry on inappropriate research and teaching; they are too expansion-oriented; and they engage in wasteful rivalry rather than in effective price competition. State and local hospitals, on the other hand, which often exist primarily to serve the poor or those who cannot obtain admission elsewhere, are frequently accused of being inefficient, hamstrung by red tape, and insensitive to patient needs.

No definitive studies of the effects of type of ownership on hospital performance are available, although American Hospital Association data permit a few broad descriptive generalizations. Proprietary hospitals tend to be small. Their average size is 74 beds compared with 182 for private nonprofit institutions. More than 80 percent of the for-profit beds are in small hospitals; the balance, with the exception of one 507-bed hospital, are in the 200–500-bed category. There are also many small state and local government hospitals — half their beds are in the under–200-bed category. There are, however, many large ones as well: one-fourth of the state and local government beds are in hospitals larger than 500 beds.

Many of the small proprietary hospitals are located in rural areas where there isn't enough community support to start a nonprofit one. Others are located in large cities or surrounding suburbs, and were typically started by groups of physicians who lacked admitting privileges at existing nonprofit hospitals. In recent years several large corporations have constructed chains of for-profit hospitals purely as commercial ventures.

The contention that the for-profit hospitals offer relatively limited facilities and services has only limited validity if one takes account of hospital size. At any given size there does not seem to be a marked difference in availability of services by type of ownership, except for psychiatric services and various kinds of outpatient services.

In each size class the occupancy rates are lower in state and local government hospitals than in either of the other types. One reasonable inference is that the public institutions are not the preferred ones in most communities. Indeed, the popular image of the public hospital is often one of limited staff and poor service to patients. The poor-service image may be justified, but it cannot be blamed on any difference in number of personnel. The AHA data reveal that for any given hospital size the number of personnel per patient is as high in the state and local government hospitals as in the private nonprofit ones. Personnel mix, however, is apparently different in the public hospitals: average earnings tend to be lower in them, for any given hospital size, than in private nonprofit hospitals. Average earnings tend to be highest in the for-profit hospitals. The difference in earnings suggests that the nonprofit hospitals, especially the publicly owned ones, may be erring in the direction of employing too many relatively low-skill personnel instead of striving for greater efficiency with fewer but better-qualified employees.

The U.S. hospital industry reveals striking regional differences that are worthy of close attention. If we understood the reasons for these differences and their consequences, we would be in a much better position to formulate rational and responsible policies for health care. The average hospital size in the West (119 beds) is much smaller than in the rest of the country — probably because of the lower population densities in the West — while average size in the Northeast (217 beds) is the largest of any region.* In keeping with the size differential, occupancy rates tend to be lowest in the West (70 percent) and highest in the Northeast (82 percent). The for-profit hospitals are relatively more important in the West (representing 12 percent of all beds) and are also somewhat important in the South (10 percent). They are much less important in the Northeast (5 percent) and almost nonexistent in the North Central region. There is also a significant regional difference in the relative importance of state and local government hospitals: they are most common in the South, accounting for 35 percent of all hospital beds there, and least common in the Northeast, where they account for 13 percent.

Probably the most striking regional difference is with respect to length of stay. In the Northeast the average patient stay is 9.2 days; in the West it is only 6.7 days. A small part of this differential — about 0.1 day — can be attributed to the difference in age composition of the population: the Northeast has a slightly older population (in 1970 10.6 percent of its population was 65 or over, as compared with 8.9 percent in the West), and older people everywhere tend to have longer stays. The differential of 2.5 days per patient, however, is far greater than can be explained by differences in age alone. At given ages and for given diagnoses, stays are significantly shorter in the West. Nor can this be explained by greater pressure for beds in that region; as has been mentioned, occupancy rates are actually lowest in the West.

In recent years hospital expenditures per capita in the Northeast have averaged 50 percent higher than in the South and 30 percent higher than in the West. The Northeast-West differential can be explained entirely by the difference in length of stay. The admission rate and expenditures per patient-day are actually slightly higher in the West than in the Northeast. The South also has significantly shorter lengths of stay than the Northeast, but this is offset in part by a higher admission rate. The major reason for the large Northeast-South cost differential is labor cost. Payroll per patient-day in the Northeast is 40 percent higher than in the South, mostly because average earnings are much higher.

---

*This discussion of regions is based on the Bureau of the Census classification of Northeast, North Central, South, and West.

TEACHING HOSPITALS

Approximately fifteen hundred hospitals in the United States are known as "teaching" hospitals, and of this number approximately nine hundred are affiliated with a medical school. These are the great medical centers which pride themselves on being able to provide the most advanced diagnostic and therapeutic services which comprise the so-called tertiary care. Most of them in fact do a superb job in teaching young physicians how to deliver that type of care. In these centers there is also considerable emphasis on research — extending the frontiers of medical practice.

Because only a small and selected fraction of persons needing or seeking health care actually enter a university-affiliated hospital, however, students there often receive a distorted view of what the health problems of the population actually are and what medicine can or should do about them. As Dr. John H. Knowles has written, "Our teaching hospitals are called health centers today when, in reality, they enjoy a limited and exclusive function as the citadels of acute curative, scientific and technical medicine."[4] John Millis, in his incisive study of medical education, notes that about three-fourths of the country's interns and residents are in university-affiliated hospitals, but that "the university has never acknowledged any responsibility for them." He calls this the "strangest anomaly in medical education" and "finds it difficult to see any rationality in this arrangement."[5] Moreover, some six hundred "teaching" hospitals that provide training for the other 25 percent of interns and residents have no university affiliation at all.

In the opinion of most experts, internship and residency training has more influence over physicians' subsequent careers than does their medical school education. The nature and quality of these programs, therefore, should be a source of considerable concern. According to some critics, the present training programs do not give future physicians a balanced view of what health care is all about because their contacts are primarily with the hospitalized patient. Interns and residents develop disdain for the ambulatory patient, for the patient with only a minor illness, for the patient with emotional and psychological problems. The young physician develops the view that the hospital is *the* place to practice medicine, a "repair shop" view of medical care that tends to crowd out the ideals of preserving and enhancing health in the community.

All too frequently hospitals have viewed interns and residents as a cheap source of labor for the delivery of care in emergency rooms and for the coverage of patients of the attending physicians. Now that salaries for interns and residents have increased appreciably, some hospitals will re-examine the desirability of maintaining such so-called teaching programs, and some will probably drop this activity.

From the resident's point of view there is a real conflict between a desire to extend one's knowledge and experience and the immediate needs of patients. I personally know of one resident who left a hospital at the midpoint of a two-year residency because he found to his dismay that the hospital was primarily interested in patient care, not in teaching. A further complication has arisen because of the disappearance of charity patients, the so-called teaching material. It is obviously desirable to have young physicians learn in actual care settings, and therefore teaching institutions will have to work out appropriate procedures so that all patients admitted can become part of the educational experience.

While there is some danger that patient needs tend to be subordinated to the research and teaching interests of the medical staff, the opposite type of problem has also arisen, particularly in large cities. I have in mind the attempts to divert medical schools from their primary responsibilities of the transmission and discovery of knowledge — teaching and research — to the delivery of services. Politicians frequently attempt to buy medical care for the poor at bargain prices by using the titles that a medical school can provide in order to hire physicians for less than they would have to pay in a strictly service setting. There can be no question that the provision of some patient care, and particularly a wide variety of services, is desirable for a medical school. But this is principally because it helps the schools to fulfill properly their primary functions of teaching and research. If government insists on emphasizing current delivery of services, however, future medical care will be imperiled.

DIRECTIONS OF CHANGE

Although we still have a long way to go, considerable progress has been made in bringing the average hospital size closer to the desirable range. Over the past twenty years the average number of beds per hospital has increased by 50 percent. The average size of for-profit hospitals, which were and are the smallest, has more than doubled. There has also been a constant upward trend in the number of hospital employees per patient, which has grown at about 2.5 percent annually for over twenty years and shows no sign of leveling off. Growth of staff is partly attributable to shortening of hours (at one time nurses worked twelve-hour days, so only two shifts were necessary) and partly to the growing complexity of hospital care. Curiously, this growth has been accompanied by increasing patient complaints about lack of service and attention. If such complaints are justified, one may well ask what all the additional staff are doing. Part of the answer must be that they are staffing and servicing the vastly more elaborate equipment now found in hospitals. The amount of capital investment per patient has been rising even more rapidly than the number of employees, and, unlike many other industries in which physical capital tends to diminish labor requirements, most new developments in medicine have tended to increase them.

Another significant trend has been the growth in importance of outpatient care. From 1962 to 1971 the number of outpatient visits more than doubled, while the number of inpatient admissions increased by only 25 percent. The surge in outpatient visits is related to the problem of access discussed in the preceding chapter. Many families no longer have a "family doctor," someone to whom they instinctively turn in time of trouble. The hospital, despite its impersonal character, is at least *there,* a known quantity where care is always accessible, albeit after a long wait. In many communities the hospital emergency room is becoming the principal source of primary care, although inpatients are still the main source of gross revenue for community hospitals, yielding about 90 percent of the total. The relative contribution of outpatient care to *net revenue,* however, is frequently significant because it tends to be more profitable than inpatient care.

The hospital industry has been expanding at an enormous rate. Employment in 1971 was twice that in 1955; in many cities one out of every twenty-five employed persons now works in a hospital. Hospital employees traditionally have not been organized, but unions have made considerable progress in hospitals in recent years, and average earnings have increased faster than the national average. These and related changes will be discussed in more detail in the next section on hospital costs.

Why Are Hospital Costs So High?

The reasons that hospital care costs so much today are complex and hard to pin down. Part of the problem is the matter of definitions: exactly what, for instance, comprises "costs"? Much of the popular discussion has focused on the cost of individual cases, noting especially how easily some patients can incur bills of five or ten thousand dollars or even more. Insofar as recent technological advances have created opportunities for treating previously untreatable conditions, high bills like these are often for procedures, such as organ transplants, that weren't possible ten or twenty years ago. As noted in Chapter 1, while the possibility of incurring such high bills is a good argument for carrying health insurance — indeed, perhaps carrying such insurance should be compulsory — it does not pose as serious a problem for analysis or policy formation as one would gather from the attention lavished on it by the popular press.

Another target the press singles out in its coverage of health care problems is high average cost per patient-day. Newspaper headlines warn that the average cost of semiprivate hospital accommodations now exceeds a hundred dollars a day and is projected to soar to two hundred dollars a day by 1980. Such emphasis on cost per day is often misplaced. Suppose, for instance, that it were possible to appreciably shorten the average length of stay. This might be highly desirable both in terms of economics and health, even though it resulted in an increase in cost per patient-day. Or suppose it were possible to reduce the number of hospital admissions by providing more ambulatory care and home nursing services. The result might be an increase in cost per patient-day for those who were admitted (because a higher percentage would be seriously ill) but a substantial decrease in total hospital costs.

Every individual has a stake in keeping the *total* as low as possible, consistent with health needs, because these costs are eventually borne by every individual — in insurance premiums and taxes if not in direct personal expenditures.

While cost per patient-day has indeed been rising rapidly, more important is the fact that total expenditures in community hospitals are now triple what they were in 1965 and more than four times the 1960 level. Some of this increase in hospital expenditures is inevitable, given that wages and prices have been increasing in the economy as a whole. The hospital industry could hardly escape paying such increases for necessary goods and services, including labor services. But if that were all that were happening the increase in hospital expenditures per capita might have been about 4 percent annually. The fact that expenditures were actually increasing at more than triple that rate is what requires special explanation.

The explanation can proceed at two levels. First, at the purely mechanical or *accounting* level it is possible statistically to break down hospital expenditures into their various components — admissions, length of stay, personnel per patient, etc. Second, one can attempt a *behavioral analysis* of patients, physicians, and others whose decisions in the aggregate determine hospital expenditures. In either case, it is also possible — and indeed, it is important — to examine rising costs over different time periods, for while hospital expenditures per capita have been rising somewhat faster than expenditures for all services ever since World War II, the differential widened enormously after 1965. Much of the hospital cost "crisis" dates from that time.

From 1950 until 1965 per capita expenditures of community hospitals grew fairly steadily at a rate of about 8 percent annually, while the figure for all services in the U.S. economy for the same period was only 5 percent annually. In the early years a good part of this differential was attributable to sharp increases in the number of personnel per patient and to wage increases that exceeded those in the general economy. This may have been a true "catching up" period for hospital employees, who prior to World War II typically worked very long hours at very low wages. The period of most rapid growth in both personnel per patient and earnings per employee was from 1950 to 1955.

Around 1960 *non*labor expenditures such as for equipment and supplies started to grow more rapidly than labor expenditures, and the average length of stay, which had been falling, started to increase. It seems to me that these changes were associated with the character of medical advances.[6] In the early post-World War II years these advances mostly took the form of new drugs that were highly effective against infectious diseases and were relatively inexpensive to administer. After 1960 many of the advances involved complex diagnostic and therapeutic procedures that were expensive and frequently resulted in longer patient stays. Between 1960 and 1965 nonlabor expenditures per admission in constant dollars grew at 7 percent annually, compared with an annual rate of only 3 percent over the 1950–1955 period.

After 1965 hospital expenditures started to explode. Between 1965 and 1971 per capita expenditures grew at approximately 14 percent annually — a rate that amounts to a doubling every five years! Service expenditures in the economy as a whole during this period grew at only 7 percent annually.

It is possible, in an accounting sense, to pinpoint the principal elements in this runaway hospital inflation. First, it should be emphasized that it was *not* due to an unusual increase in the number of patients. Patient-days per capita grew at about the same rate after 1965 as before. Second, expenditures for labor and especially for nonlabor inputs per patient-day grew exceptionally rapidly. The number of personnel per patient after 1965 jumped by 3.4 percent annually, compared with a 1.7 percent annual rate from 1960 to 1965. Earnings per employee after 1965 soared at 8 percent annually. By contrast, earnings for all workers in the private nonagricultural economy grew at less than 5 percent annually during these same years. The sharp increase in nonlabor expenditures went mostly for new and more elaborate equipment and for supplies, including more disposables and prepared-prepackaged food.

Turning to a behavioral explanation of these same phenomena, a rich variety of hypotheses present themselves. One of the most compelling is that 1966 marked the introduction of Medicare and Medicaid, two large federal health insurance programs that made available huge amounts of new money for hospital care. The resulting large increase in demand for services was relatively insensitive to higher prices, because reimbursement was geared to cost. According to Professor Herbert Klarman, a leading authority on the economics of hospitals, the volume of services reimbursed on a cost basis jumped 75 percent as a result of the establishment of Medicare and Medicaid.[7]

This created an unprecedented opportunity for physicians and hospital administrators to do what they always want to do — improve the quality of care as they see it. This means more equipment, more personnel, more tests, more X rays, and so on. It did not, as noted above, result in an abnormal increase in the number of people getting care, but the intensity of care increased appreciably. The big unknown in the equation is: what effect, if any, has this had on health? Were physicians and hospital administrators truly serving the social interest, or were they merely fulfilling their own "technological imperative"? Was there a divergence between their interests and those of the community, or did they improperly diagnose the community's health needs and the consequences of the decisions they were making?

One reasonable interpretation is that the physician who pressed for more equipment and staff in the hospital was doing what was regarded as best for the patient, since the patient would get some benefit while the costs would be passed on to a third party (i.e., the federal government). The collective effect of these individual decisions, however, was what many regard as an unwarranted increase in the cost of hospital care. Unfortunately, this large increase in resources devoted to hospital care does not seem to have produced improvement in the health of the population. Whether in the absence of this increase there would have been deterioration in health is a matter for further conjecture and study.

A case study by Professor Bernard Friedman of the treatment of breast cancer in six Boston hospitals provides a possible illustration of the process described above. In 1965, prior to the introduction of Medicare and Medicaid, about 20 percent of the cases were treated with both surgery and radiation; the other 80 percent of cases received only one or the other treatment, at least initially. In 1967 more than 40 percent of (apparently similar) cases received initial treatment of both surgery and radiation. Friedman is not certain that the change in treatment was due to Medicare. He notes that women under age 65 also experienced changes in treatment, but speculates that this may be partly the result of a Medicare-induced change in the "standard" of care. It would be nice to be able to say that the additional care had a positive impact on survival, but Friedman reports that the percentage of patients who died within three years of initial treatment was essentially the same before and after Medicare.[8]

How to Keep Hospital Costs from Going Higher

Rufus Rorem, who did pioneering studies of health economics nearly fifty years ago, said that one of the most widely read articles he ever wrote was entitled "Why Hospital Costs Have Risen." The demand for reprints was enormous. Encouraged by this success he then wrote an article entitled "How to Keep Hospital Costs From Rising." Judging from a complete lack of requests, this piece was a total failure.

Rorem's experience is indicative of an attitude that was and perhaps still is all too common in the health field. Shrouded in the mantle of "nonprofit" and convinced of the worthiness of all their endeavors, hospital administrations have been primarily concerned with justifying high costs rather than considering whether the resources siphoned into the hospital field might not be better used in other directions, including other dimensions of health care. Moreover, even when administrators attempt to take a broader view, their freedom to act is sharply limited by the hospital's physicians on the one hand and the board of trustees on the other.

An approach to the control of hospital expenditures can profitably begin with a simple definition:

$$\text{Expenditures} = \text{Admissions} \times \text{Length of stay} \times \text{Cost per patient-day}$$

There is no way to affect hospital expenditures except by altering one or more of these variables.

Admissions

Hospital admissions per capita in the United States have been rising fairly steadily ever since 1950 at a bit over 1 percent annually. At present one out of every seven Americans enters a community hospital as an in-patient each year, while in 1950 only one in every nine did. If the present trend continues, by the end of the century the rate will be one out of every five. Inasmuch as it is doubtful that there is more morbidity in the population now than there used to be, it is not clear why admission rates have been rising.

One school of thought holds that the rate of admissions responds to bed availability: if we insist on installing more hospital beds, they will tend to get filled. This proposition, dubbed "Roemer's law," after Dr. Milton Roemer of UCLA, who first suggested it in 1959, has received considerable support in recent econometric studies.

The notion that supply can create its own demand in this market should not come as too much of a surprise. The decision to admit or discharge patients is largely in the hands of the physician. Such decisions are supposedly made on scientific grounds, but medical science is not exact and there are many cases where a plausible argument can be made either way. In such instances the availability or lack of availability of a bed can have a significant influence on the decision.

Many physicians have a built-in bias in favor of hospitalization. As mentioned previously, their training is heavily oriented toward the hospitalized patient. When in doubt they feel more comfortable if the patient is in the hospital. It is more convenient for the physician, there is more control and supervision of the patient's condition, it is easier to carry on diagnostic work, and emergency care is more readily available if needed.

One obvious way, therefore, to hold down hospital admissions is to sharply limit the expansion in the number of hospital beds. Such limitation can be sought through government regulation, by curtailing federal funding for new construction, or, as discussed below, by changing hospital reimbursement plans so as to eliminate the guarantee that the hospital will always be able to meet its bills.

From the patient's point of view hospital admission frequently seems attractive even when not medically necessary because one's insurance will pay for procedures done as an inpatient but not as an outpatient. Another strategy, therefore, is to modify health insurance plans so that they do not encourage such inappropriate use of facilities. Adding outpatient coverage would tend to eliminate some hospital admissions, but it may also result in an increase in total health expenditures. A great deal depends on incentives offered physicians. Prepaid group practices such as the Kaiser health plans have demonstrated that it is possible to reduce substantially hospital admission rates without drastically increasing outpatient visits or jeopardizing patient health. Such plans have recorded admission rates one-third to one-half lower than those for comparable populations with conventional insurance coverage. A significant amount of the difference is related to the lower rates of in-hospital surgery among members of prepaid plans.

Some observers believe that the key factor in such plans is the financial incentive given to physicians to hold down hospital utilization; in some of the Kaiser plans the physicians benefit when hospital costs fall below projected levels. Others believe that the key is to be found in the limited availability of hospital beds. Because the number of beds per capita is often half of what is considered a "normal" ratio, Kaiser physicians are forced to reconsider the appropriate decision for a large number of marginal conditions.

Still others believe that the lower admissions under such plans can be attributed to the free or nearly free care available to outpatients, which results in much less pressure from patients for hospitalization. As has been stated, however, it does not appear that the reduced use of hospitals under such plans is accomplished by an unusual increase in outpatient care. My own view is that the capitation method of payment is the critical variable in changing physician behavior: when physicians know that there is only so much money available and that extra spending in the hospital has implications for the rest of the plan, they tend to use hospitals much more judiciously.

Length of Stay

Once a patient is admitted to the hospital there can be considerable variation in the length of stay, with significant implications for hospital expenditures. An important determinant is the efficiency with which the staff carries out the necessary diagnostic and therapeutic procedures. Are there delays in conducting tests and taking X rays? Do these have to be repeated because of errors? Are operating rooms available when needed? Do patients linger longer than necessary simply because their physicians are away or have forgotten to discharge them? Adverse side effects of drugs, tests, and surgery also frequently increase the length of stay. One study of hospitalization for neurosurgery found that postoperative infection, which occurred in 17 percent of the cases, extended the average stay (twenty-five days) by an additional eighteen days.[9]

The length of stay that physicians deem appropriate for various medical conditions often has a weak scientific basis. The few studies that have been done suggest that considerable variation is possible without discernible health effects. In England, for instance, a controlled study of patients who had been operated on for hernia could find no significant differences between patients who were discharged one day after surgery and comparable patients who were discharged after six days.[10]

Dr. Paul T. Lahti, a surgeon who is a vigorous advocate of early hospital discharge after surgery, contends that such procedure is actually better for the patient's health. Lahti has reported that of 611 consecutive patients on whom he performed a variety of general surgical procedures — including herniorrhaphies, appendectomies, and cholecystectomies (surgical excision of the gall bladder) — only 21 percent stayed in the hospital four days or more. The largest percentage went home on the first post-operative day.[11] Most physicians who perform the same type of surgery as Dr. Lahti keep their patients in the hospital about four or five days longer.

Length of stay for nonsurgical cases is also frequently arbitrary and lacking in scientific basis. A prospective controlled study of 138 randomly selected patients with uncomplicated but definite myocardial infarction tested the proposition that patients discharged after two weeks of hospital stay can do as well as those discharged after three weeks. For six months after discharge (as far as the study went) there appeared to be no additional benefit to the patients who received the three-week stay.[12]

A critical factor to consider before discharging a patient from the hospital before complete recovery is the nature and amount of care available on the outside. Sometimes all that is needed is an occasional visit by a nurse, or someone to provide a hot meal, or a conveniently located outpatient facility. Sometimes a simpler, less expensive type of institution, such as an extended-care facility, is indicated.

Even when such facilities are available, however, there may be institutional barriers that prolong hospitalization unnecessarily. Dr. Sidney Lee cites the example of a hospital that was planning to expand, because of pressure on capacity, even though an attached extended-care facility was half-empty. It was discovered that physicians were reluctant to transfer patients from the hospital to the attached facility because they had to complete a lengthy form and because the third party did not cover physician services in the facility. Simplification of the form and a change in the third-party coverage provisions put an end to plans for hospital expansion and resulted in significant savings in total health care costs.[13]

A legitimate concern of physicians who might otherwise be willing to consider earlier discharge is whether they can get their patients promptly readmitted in an emergency. Arrangements for such contingencies are certainly feasible, but in the absence of more concrete incentives for administrator, physician, and patient, early discharge is not likely to come into being.

One irony of hospital economics is that longer stays help to keep down the average cost per patient-day. This happens for two reasons. First, patients who stay on after the acute phase of their illness make fewer demands on staff and equipment. Second, it is easier to maintain a high occupancy rate when there is a less rapid turnover in patients. Thus short stays make life more difficult for hospital administrators and their staffs. Most administrators want to keep their occupancy rates up, and when too many beds become unoccupied, they try to put pressure on the physicians to fill them. One way is to suggest to each of the various service chiefs (for medicine, surgery, pediatrics, etc.) that unless they keep the beds assigned to their respective service reasonably full they will be reassigned to another service. The result is a tendency to admit more freely and especially to have longer stays.

Attempts at controlling length of stay have been made both through internal review in the hospital and by third-party payers. In many areas of the country, for example, the Blue Cross plan keeps records on the average length of stay in each hospital for each diagnosis and exerts some pressure on hospitals and on physicians by asking them to justify unusually long stays. Of course, if hospitals were reimbursed in part on the number of cases treated rather than only the number of days of care rendered this would provide a stronger and more direct incentive for shorter stays.

Cost per Patient-Day

Given hospital admission rates and average lengths of stay, the only way to control expenditures — as the equation on page 96 indicates — is by reducing the cost per patient-day. About 60 percent of this cost now goes for labor and about 40 percent for nonlabor inputs. This total cost may exceed the socially optimal level in a given hospital for three reasons. First, given the fact that resources are needed for other pressing social needs, the hospital may be providing "too much" service or care. Second, it may be providing its services inefficiently, that is, using too many resources. And finally, it may be paying too high a price for the goods and services (including labor) that it buys. In most areas of the economy we rely on management's hope of profit and fear of loss to avoid such errors. With respect to hospitals it might be possible to introduce similar incentives by instituting new methods of reimbursement.

INCENTIVE REIMBURSEMENT

Reimbursement of hospitals in the aggregate clearly must bear some relationship to costs. If not, the hospital system would dissolve for failure to command the resources necessary to stay in business. But it does not follow that the reimbursement formula must permit each and every hospital to stay in business, nor does it follow that each service maintained by a hospital should have *its* full cost reimbursed regardless of its social utility.

One proposal for monitoring hospital costs would require each hospital to justify its annual budget to third-party payers or to a regulatory agency. Such a line-by-line policing of hospital decisions, where the judgment of the reviewer is presumably substituted for that of the hospital administration, would probably be difficult and expensive to administer and over time would tend to become very inflexible.

An alternative approach that I have advocated[14] provides considerable incentive for efficient management, permits great flexibility, and is administratively much more simple. The starting point of this approach is average cost (ideally both cost per case and cost per patient-day would be used) for all community hospitals. Statistical analysis would be used to determine the effect on cost of location, services offered, and various other hospital characteristics. The reimbursement rate for each hospital would then be established as a function of the average cost of all hospitals combined adjusted for the characteristics of the particular hospital. Thus hospitals located in higher wage areas, or those offering more services, would get above-average reimbursement; those in low-wage areas or offering fewer services would get less.

While statistical analysis could be used as a starting point to determine adjustments for different services, there is no reason why the third-party reimburser could not raise (or lower) the adjustment factor for particular services that it wished to encourage (or discourage). For instance, analysis might show that, other things being equal, the presence of an open-heart surgery facility adds two dollars to the patient-day cost of an average hospital. If the third party deemed this a poor use of resources, it could lower the adjustment factor to one dollar per patient-day. Hospitals so affected would thus have considerable incentive to eliminate this service, especially if it were infrequently used. On the other hand, if the third party desired to encourage hospitals to have certain services, say intensive-care units, it could raise the adjustment factor for this service. In contrast to reimbursement schemes where a central bureaucracy makes all the decisions, this system leaves a good deal of discretion to individual hospitals. Thus the judgment, experience, knowledge of local needs, and creative intelligence of physicians and administrators throughout the country would be allowed considerable scope.

One big advantage of this approach is that no hospital administration could be certain in advance that all its costs would be met. Thus an administration would be under constant pressure to keep costs in check while still meeting patient and physician demands for care. In describing this plan to hospital administrators I have always received the same reaction: each one is convinced that the respective hospital would get less reimbursement under this plan than it now gets. This is curious, since the plan, including the adjustments, calls for reimbursing in the aggregate the full cost of the system. The fact that each administrator fears the effect of such a plan on the respective hospital speaks volumes about the potential for eliminating waste and inefficiency.

This system, which appears to put hospital administrators under greater pressure, would, paradoxically, strengthen their position *vis-à-vis* the physicians. Under direct cost reimbursement an administrator finds it difficult to refuse requests for more equipment or staff regardless of one's opinion of their cost effectiveness: a service chief can always tell the administrator that when costs rise, so will the rate of reimbursement. But if there were a real possibility that the hospital would not be able to meet its bills, the administrator's "no" would carry a great deal more conviction and authority.

One disadvantage of such a system is that the hospital administration might be tempted to skimp on the services and care provided to patients. Some "skimping" is obviously what is wanted, but protection against unwarranted risks to patient health or safety would have to depend on the vigilance of physicians, accreditation bodies, third-party purchasers, and patients.

COMPETITION OR REGULATION?

I am much in favor of trying to introduce more competitive behavior into the hospital field through the reimbursement mechanism, but I doubt that the industry can be safely left to a pure free-market approach. The essence of a free competitive market is that (1) there are many well-informed buyers and sellers no one of whom is large enough to influence price unilaterally; (2) buyers and sellers act independently (i.e., there is no collusion); and (3) there is free entry for other buyers and sellers not currently in the market. Many hospital markets depart substantially from these ideal competitive conditions, sometimes inevitably.

In most towns and even moderate-size cities the market is too small to support enough hospitals to fulfill the requirements of free competition. As was pointed out previously, there are significant economies of scale in hospitals up to a size of at least 200 or 300 beds. Since a community needs no more than 4 beds per 1,000 population (and probably less), a city of 60,000 would be most efficiently served by a single well-run hospital. It would thus be uneconomical to require numerous competitive hospitals except in large, densely populated markets. These constraints are even more imperative when specialty care is considered. It is doubtful that a population even as large as 1 million justifies enough independent maternity, open-heart surgery, and organ-transplant services to provide really competitive conditions. The fact that these services proliferate contrary to what economies of scale would indicate is the result of other problems, such as the absence of appropriate incentives and constraints for physicians and hospital administrators.

In such a condition of "natural monopoly" the traditional American response has been to introduce public utility regulation (e.g., electric utility, telephone, transportation). The results, however, have frequently been unsatisfactory, partly because the regulators often tend to serve the regulated rather than the public and partly because it is inherently difficult to set standards of performance without competitive yardsticks. Many other countries rely on government ownership and control, but the United States experience with government hospitals has not, on balance, been favorable. Another possible solution is the development of what J. K. Galbraith has termed "countervailing power" and what the economics textbooks describe as "bilateral monopoly." If, for instance, all the consumers in a one-hospital town were organized into a single body for purposes of bargaining with the hospital, at least some of the disadvantages of monopoly would be lessened.

The typical "solution" in the hospital field has been to emphasize the "nonprofit" character of community hospitals and to assume that because of it they will not abuse their monopoly power. This "solution" is open to the criticisms that the absence of a profit (loss) incentive too easily leads to waste, inefficiency, and unnecessary duplication and that perhaps the hospitals are run for the benefit of the physicians.

Even when there are numerous hospitals in the same market, society may benefit if they refrain from maintaining arm's-length competitive postures with one another. The free exchange of information, cooperative efforts to meet crisis situations, and reciprocal backup arrangements may help to reduce costs and increase patient satisfaction. Unfortunately, the intimacy and trust developed through such activities may spread in less desirable directions such as price fixing, exclusion of would-be rivals, and other practices restricting competition. For two hundred years economists have been impressed with the wisdom of Adam Smith's observation in *The Wealth of Nations* that "people of the same trade seldom meet together, even for merriment and diversion, but the conversation ends in a conspiracy against the public, or in some contrivance to raise prices."

Although some deviation from a purely competitive solution seems inevitable, regulation of hospitals by state public utility commissions would, in my opinion, be a disaster. In the first place, our experience with other industries has taught us that regulation is frequently introduced at the behest of the regulated as a device for achieving legal cartelization and restricting competition. Hospitals would certainly be no exception to this rule. The leading proponent of state public utility regulation approach is the American Hospital Association. Second, experience has shown that regulation rarely works to lower prices and frequently results in inefficiency and undesirable costs. Finally, regulation would tend to inhibit technological and organizational innovation.[15]

Public utility commissions, even if well managed by well-motivated men and women, would inevitably concentrate on setting per diem prices (based on cost) rather than on looking at the total cost of care to the community. The person who is in the best position to exert intelligent restraints on hospital costs is the physician. The physician knows better than anyone which patients need not be admitted, which ones could go home a day earlier, which tests are really superfluous. The physician is also best situated to appraise the excess capacity now appearing in many hospital care markets. When one considers that perhaps one out of every five patients now in a hospital need not be there, the possibility of really serious overcapacity cannot be lightly dismissed. As a first step toward getting a grip on hospital costs, a five-year moratorium should be declared (allowing very few exceptions) on all hospital construction and expansion. During this period the financing system should be modified so as to provide incentives to physicians and hospital administrators and trustees to balance costs against potential benefits. With hospital costs under control, more funds would be available for ambulatory care, preventive medicine, treatment of emotional problems, medical research, and other needs that are currently being squeezed out of the picture by our resource-devouring hospital system.

Supplementary Reading

Please see "How To Save $1 Trillion Out of Health Care" in Part 2.

CHAPTER 5

Drugs: The Key
to Modern Medicine

> Powerful drugs are a mixed blessing. Active
> chemicals inevitably carry with them the
> capacity for both good and harm.
>
> LOUIS LASAGNA, M.D.
> "Research Regulation and Development
> of New Pharmaceuticals: Past, Present
> and Future," *The American Journal of
> the Medical Sciences*

Drugs are the key to modern medicine. Surgery, radiotherapy, and diagnostic tests are all important, but the ability of health care providers to alter health outcomes — Dr. Walsh McDermott's "decisive technology" — depends primarily on drugs. Six dollars are spent on hospitals and physicians for every dollar spent on drugs, but without drugs the effectiveness of hospitals and physicians would be enormously diminished.

The great power of drugs is a development of the twentieth century — many would say of the past forty years. Our age has been given many names — atomic, electronic, space, and the like — but measured by impact on people's lives it might just as well be called the "drug age."

Until this century the physician could with confidence give a smallpox vaccination, administer quinine for malaria, prescribe opium and morphine for the relief of pain, and not much more. As Dr. Allen Norton has noted, "The decades around 1900 were a time of famous diagnosticians. The cynic could reasonably say that this was not surprising. There was no other way in which an able doctor could express himself because there were so few remedies for any diseases."[1]

A quarter-century later the situation was not much different. Some advances had been made in surgery, but the death rates from tuberculosis, influenza and pneumonia, and other infectious diseases were still extremely high. With the introduction and wide use of sulfonamide and penicillin, however, the death rate in the

United States from influenza and pneumonia fell by more than 8 percent annually from 1935 to 1950. (The annual rate of decline from 1900 to 1935 had been only 2 percent.) In the case of tuberculosis, while some progress had been made since the turn of the century, the rate of decline in the death rate accelerated appreciably after the adoption of penicillin, streptomycin, and PAS (paraaminosalicylic acid) in the late 1940s and of isoniazid in the early 1950s. New drugs and vaccines developed since the 1920s have also been strikingly effective against typhoid, whooping cough, poliomyelitis, measles, diphtheria, and tetanus; more recently great advances have been made in hormonal drugs, antihypertension drugs, antihistamines, anticoagulants, antipsychotic drugs, and antidepressants.

The great scientific advances of this century have been matched by a rapid growth in the size of the drug industry. In 1899, the year that marked the introduction of aspirin, the U.S. drug industry had a value added by manufacture* of just over $50 million. By 1929 this figure had increased sixfold, and the industry's most rapid expansion was yet to come. Between 1939 and 1958, a period when many of today's most effective drugs were introduced and widely diffused for the first time, the industry's value added multiplied eightfold, while that of manufacturing as a whole increased by less than six times. By 1970 the value added of the drug industry was over $5 *billion* dollars, making it one of the largest manufacturing industries in the country. (Only the motor vehicle, aircraft, iron and steel, industrial chemicals, and communications equipment industries have appreciably larger value added.)

Given its economic importance, its rapid rate of growth, and the unique contribution of some of its output to human welfare, it should be no surprise that the drug industry has begun to receive a great deal of attention from lawmakers, the press, and some academic researchers. The topics that have provoked greatest interest are drug safety, overuse and abuse of drugs, drug prices, drug industry profits, drug advertising, and drug research. Discussion of these topics and the policy issues that surround them follows a description of the drug industry.

Drug Manufacturing

About one thousand U.S. firms are engaged in the manufacture of drugs. Most of these firms are small, limiting their attention either to manufacturing a few specialized products, or to serving local areas, or to repackaging drugs bought in bulk from other producers. About one hundred firms, members of the Pharmaceutical Manufacturers Association, account for most of the industry's production, including about 95 percent of prescription drug sales. Prescription

---

*The *value added by manufacture* for a given industry is defined as the value of its shipments minus the cost of materials and supplies purchased from other industries.

drugs are much more important than nonprescription ("over-the-counter") drugs from both the medical and economic points of view, and their relative importance has been increasing. Several U.S. drug firms are worldwide in scope, with from one-fourth to one-half of their production and sales taking place outside the United States. Conversely, about 10 to 15 percent of domestic drug consumption is produced by American subsidiaries of foreign companies.

Academic economists, in appraising the drug or any industry, typically attach paramount importance to its structure, by which they mean the size distribution of firms. Do a few large firms account for most of the industry's sales, or are there many effective competitors? Economic theory suggests (and historical experience confirms) that if the former is true, collusion among the dominant firms to fix prices and the practice of other kinds of restrictive and monopolistic behavior are more likely to occur. Explicit collusion (secret meetings and agreements to fix prices) is much easier to manage when only a handful of firms are involved, as is implicit collusion (setting one's prices in line with major competitors' prices in order to keep profits at satisfactorily high levels).

A commonly used index of "concentration" (a term denoting the size distribution of firms) is the proportion of industry output accounted for by the four largest (or eight largest) firms. For the U.S. drug industry this index is not exceptionally high. The four largest firms account for about 25 percent of all output, the eight largest for less than 50 percent — somewhat lower than typical figures for other U.S. chemical or manufacturing industries, and much lower than the indexes for the American automobile, aircraft, iron and steel, and many other industries.

There is, however, something special about drug manufacturing which makes the concentration index for the industry less relevant than usual. The output of most drug firms is specialized, with no possibility of substituting drugs in one category for those in another. Major product categories like antihistamines, antiinfectives, tranquilizers, cardiovascular preparations, and gastrointestinal preparations cannot compete with one another for sales the way that Chryslers compete with Chevrolets or even the way phonograph records compete with tapes. Thus to get a true picture of the drug industry's competitive structure one must calculate separate concentration indexes by product category. And these are typically quite high. In most instances the top four firms account for 50 to 60 percent of sales. Contributing to this lack of competition within drug product categories is the fact that production techniques for different types of drug products often differ considerably. Thus even the potential ability of drug firms to compete across product categories is sometimes limited — when not actually barred by patents — by lack of process "know-how" and of specialized production facilities.

Although the concentration indexes for drug product categories are at high levels, over time there is considerable turnover among category leaders. Of the top five firms in any category in a given year, there is a good chance that two or three will not be among the top five a decade later. Such turnovers, however, are usually the result of new-product development, and are rarely due to price competition.

PRICE POLICIES

In most industries, and especially in competitive ones, prices tend to fall when costs of production fall and to rise when costs rise. The prices of most prescription drugs, however, tend to remain constant for very long periods of time. Such price inflexibility, even when there have been large changes in demand and/or costs of production, suggests a remarkable freedom from competitive pressures.

While list prices tend to remain fixed for long periods, the price charged by a drug manufacturer often varies greatly depending upon the customer. Differences have been reported of as much as 500 percent between the price charged drug retailers (i.e., pharmacies) and the price charged hospitals, or between the domestic and the export price. Such differences, unless justified by equivalent differences in cost (and frequently they are not), are evidence of price discrimination. Such conduct suggests that drug manufacturers possess and use monopoly power, just as the ability of physicians to charge different fees to different patients has been taken as evidence of the weakness of competition in that market.[2]

Why do drug companies practice price discrimination? Because maximum profits are realized by cutting prices where sales are likely to be responsive to such cuts and by maintaining them in all other markets. The price discriminator makes more this way than if charging a uniform price or one that simply varied with differences in cost. In markets where there is effective price competition, however, such a policy cannot succeed.

Drug manufacturers charge lower prices to hospitals and to the buyer on the export markets because the range of possible substitutes open to both is greater than that available to either retailers or domestic buyers in general. Hospitals, for example, are in a position to negotiate with several potential suppliers; moreover, they can conduct tests to determine whether quality standards are being met. The individual drug retailer, on the other hand, must stock whatever the customers require — and what the customers require is usually determined by the physician. Export markets are more competitive than domestic markets because there is more possibility of substitution from foreign producers.

Drug industry spokespersons resent the charge that they are not competitive. From their point of view, competition is keen, but is manifest in the development of new and better drug products. Such competition, they argue, serves the consumer better than would simple price competition on existing drugs. Drug research and development is a long and expensive process, with many years usually intervening between the initiation of research and the successful marketing of a new drug product. The hope of securing a monopoly position and the profits that go with it provides the incentive for firms to undertake that process.

PRODUCT DIFFERENTIATION

One of the outstanding characteristics of the drug industry is its emphasis on product differentiation. Much of the research effort, and nearly all of the marketing effort of major firms is devoted to developing drugs that, no matter how closely they resemble other drugs, are perceived as distinctive and superior. The distinctiveness and superiority of each brand is emphasized by heavy advertising and promotional efforts that, in the case of prescription drugs, attempt to persuade physicians to prescribe that brand rather than another manufacturer's version. By making minor modifications in the chemical formula of a drug, each manufacturer can truthfully claim that one's product is "different," even though its mode of action and its effects are similar to other companies' drugs.

Distinctiveness is also sought by developing new dosage forms of existing drugs — capsules instead of tablets, an inhalant instead of a liquid, etc. — and by combining existing drugs into new products. In the 1950s such attempts at minor differentiation reached their peak. Less than 10 percent of the new drug products marketed during that decade were new chemical entities; most were combination products, new dosage forms, or simply duplications.

Every such attempt at product differentiation has some possible good consequences as well as bad ones. Physicians can prescribe reputable brand names with reasonable confidence in the uniformity and quality of the product. New dosage forms and combination products may serve the needs of some patients better than existing products. Minor molecular manipulation may result in a significant therapeutic advance: according to Dr. J. J. Burns, vice-president for research of Hoffman, LaRoche (a major drug manufacturer), "The steroids, sulfonamides, antihistamines and semi-synthetic penicillins, to cite a few types, are replete with examples of major bio-medical advancements resulting from allegedly minor molecular manipulation."[3]

On the other side of the ledger, excessive differentiation of basically similar drugs obviously results in increased prices for the consumer. Differentiation is usually accompanied by high expenditures for advertising and other sales efforts, much of it concentrated on establishing the drug's distinctiveness to a degree far beyond that which could be justified by a scientific comparison of the products in question. Another reason different versions of the same drug result in higher costs is because pharmacies must carry a larger inventory of products than is really necessary.

The advertising techniques used to promote the sale of *non*prescription drugs, as might be expected, are similar to those which are used to market cigarettes, beer, and cosmetics. What is more surprising, and disturbing, is the flashy prescription-drug advertising that appears in medical journals and is directed at physicians — professionals who presumably should not be so easily influenced by pictures of pretty girls or chic typography. In addition to advertising, U.S. drug firms employ over twenty thousand "detailers," sales persons whose primary job is to visit physicians and push their company's products.

In defense of these practices the drug companies contend, with some justification, that information about new drugs must be delivered to the physician somehow, and that there is no cost-free way of doing this under any economic or political system. This is correct. Critics of the drug industry, however, seriously question whether it is necessary to spend, as do the drug companies collectively, an average of as much as $4,000 annually on every practicing physician in the United States in order to "provide the information needed."

Not all competition among drug companies, then, takes the form of developing new drugs. Some is simply old-fashioned competition in marketing, but with the emphasis on persuasion, not price. Consider, for example, the methods of one of the country's fastest-growing drug companies as described in a 1971 *Fortune* article. Started as a one-person operation in 1950, by 1962 this firm was boasting annual sales of close to $2 million. With the help of high-pressure selling tactics, sales have since grown to over $50 million annually, while the company's founder has accumulated a personal fortune of over $150 million. The company, the *Fortune* article reports, "spends virtually nothing on basic research, it owns no patents on drugs it manufactures, and it has no products with exclusive therapeutic properties." Its salespersons, however, "make twice as many calls on doctors as salesmen from 50 leading pharmaceutical companies."[4]

Aggressive salesmanship clearly has a place in the American free-enterprise system. Neither expressions of moral outrage against the drug industry nor the passing of a flock of new laws is likely to alter the situation. The only person who can make prescribing more rational is the physician, being the only one who writes prescriptions. If the physician had a financial stake in keeping down the cost of the drugs prescribed, as someone would under a comprehensive capitation prepayment plan, the physician might be motivated to examine more closely drug prices and alternative products — and the physician undoubtedly would also be less susceptible to persuasive detailers (sales representatives) and high-pressure advertising.

Keeping abreast of drugs is not an easy task for the physician. It is obviously difficult for a busy practitioner to be familiar with the properties, prices, and potential dangers of more than a small fraction of the eight thousand drug products listed in the *Physician's Desk Reference* (a commercial publication distributed free to physicians). One physician in five tries to keep up to date by subscribing to the *Medical Letter*, a nonprofit newsletter published biweekly. In highly readable language this four-page publication reviews new drugs and new experience with old drugs, provides advice about drug interactions and other adverse effects, and also supplies the physician with price information that could result in great savings for the patient. One item in the May 11, 1973 issue, for instance, discussed the use and cost of oral penicillins. Noting that some brands cost three to four times as much as the same dose in generic form,* the item went on to point out that "there

---

*Many drugs are manufactured in generic form — i.e., without a brand name — as well as under various brand names. Thus many companies produce *penicillin* (the generic term), some of them under brand names like V-cillin (Lilly), Veetids (Squibb), and Iticillin VK (Upjohn).

is no evidence of clinically important differences in the bioavailability [a measure of quality] of oral generic and brand-name products." The same issue also cautioned against the inappropriate prescribing of ampicillin (a related drug), which in brand-name form can cost six to seven times as much as unbranded penicillin, although for many purposes it "offers no important advantage over oral penicillin" while producing "a higher incidence of skin rashes and diarrhea."[5]

Unless physicians have access to reliable information from noncommercial sources, they tend to be unduly influenced by advertisements and detailers. The problem is particularly acute for physicians who practice alone, whereas rational prescribing is facilitated in an organized group setting where each physician can more easily benefit from the experience of colleagues and where joint efforts at systematic appraisal of new drugs can be made to determine efficacy, toxicity, and cost.

Drug Retailing

About one-fourth of the drug industry's total output is sold to hospitals, governments, and other bulk buyers, while three-fourths is distributed through retail pharmacies. More than half of all the drugs sold by retailers come to them through drug wholesalers, whose markup is usually small (about 10 percent of the retail price) and covers the cost of such essential functions as storage, credit, and delivery. Unlike drug manufacturing and drug retailing, the wholesaling sector of the drug business has never seemed to pose any special problems for public policy.

The drug retailer's markup is typically about 40 to 50 percent of the selling price, although these are average figures and the actual markup can and does vary greatly. Retailers sharply disagree regarding the basic policy they should follow in charging for their services. Some apply a fixed percentage markup to every drug, while others charge a fixed dispensing fee, such as two dollars per prescription, regardless of the drug's retail price. The latter practice makes more sense from the economic point of view because the costs to the retailer that are involved in dispensing a drug are not likely to vary much or at all with the price of the drug.

There are about fifty thousand retail drugstores in the United States — or one for every four office-based physicians. About 90 percent are independently owned; the others are owned by chains. The chain stores are, on average, about five times larger than the independents, but most of the difference in size reflects sales of merchandise other than prescription drugs. The bulk of prescriptions are still dispensed by independent owner-operated pharmacies. There is, however, growing price competition from discount chains, and this competition is changing the retail drug market, especially in large cities. No one knows how significant discounting has become, but it appears that careful shopping for drugs can result in substantial savings.

According to a recent editorial in *Drug Topics,* a leading trade publication for pharmacists, some observers predict that "the quality chain drugstore and the highminded independent [are] on the way to becoming as extinct as the passenger pigeon," being driven out by "aggressive discounters." The editorial goes on to criticize the discounters for skimping on services, and concludes by recommending state-administered price controls that "would make it illegal to sell a prescription drug below a certain level."[6]

The controversies concerning drug retailing should be viewed in the context of the changing role of the pharmacist. In earlier decades, the pharmacist manufactured many of the drugs dispensed. Now the pills and liquids are usually compounded at the factory, and the production part of the pharmacist's job consists of transferring the prescribed quantity from a large jar to a smaller one. Even that task is being made unnecessary by the increasing use of prepackaged prescriptions in quantities most frequently ordered by physicians.

These trends have prompted some observers to contend that the pharmacist is overtrained for the few simple tasks one actually performs. Evidence that this is the case is fairly strong, and many large pharmacies now make extensive use of pharmacist's aides (typically high school graduates with on-the-job training). They work under the supervision of a licensed pharmacist (who ordinarily has had five years of specialized training beyond high school). There is a completely different way of viewing the situation, however. Given the potency of modern drugs to do harm as well as good, there is a need, some argue, for pharmacological experts to keep track of all the drugs their customers take, to know what drugs their customers are allergic to, to keep abreast of new drugs and new findings about old drugs (including possible adverse interactions and side effects), and to be well versed in drug costs and drug quality. It is unlikely that many pharmacists currently fulfill this role, but the need exists and, therefore, it is plausible to suggest that, in another sense, pharmacists are "undertrained."

Another controversy surrounding drug retailing today concerns the advertising of prescription drug prices by pharmacies. The traditional position is that such advertising is "unprofessional," that patients should choose their pharmacist on the basis of convenience, service, and reputation, without regard to cost. At the instigation of pharmacy owners, most states have passed laws prohibiting the advertising of prescription drug prices, although recent court decisions have called into question the constitutionality of such legislation.

Public opinion, moreover, has been aroused by the discovery that the price for the same prescription item in the same city can vary by as much as 200 to 300 percent depending upon the pharmacy selling it. Studies have also revealed that some pharmacies charge different prices for the same prescription depending on the race or social class of the customer. A few large drug chains have begun to display their prices openly, and the city of Boston, for example, *requires* drugstores to post the prices of a specified list of nearly a hundred drugs.

Drugstores do differ in the services provided. Variations in the range of stock maintained, location, store hours, credit policy, and delivery services all affect the cost of doing business. Perhaps most important from a health point of view, pharmacists differ in the extent to which they keep accurate records, note side effects and allergic reactions, and work with physicians as members of the health team.

From the economic point of view, customers should be free to buy where they think they are best served, and with as much information as possible, including price. Price, however, should not be the only consideration. The problem is, of course, greatly complicated by the fact that the patient often lacks any familiarity with the product being purchased. In many cases the physician may not have even mentioned the name of the drug prescribed.

The prescribing and taking of drugs is a critical part of the health care process. Questions about the organization of drug dispensing are best handled, in my view, by integrating them with the broader questions of the overall organization and delivery of medical care. As previously suggested, the surest way to get physicians to give more thought to their prescribing is to give them a financial stake in keeping down the cost of drugs. Capitation prepayment that includes drugs does this. Moreover, establishing a closer relationship between the pharmacist and the physician would contribute to the improvement of health care by assuring the more efficacious use of drugs and fewer adverse reactions.

New Drugs

The drugs developed in recent decades have been major factors in improving the prevention, cure, and alleviation of disease and pain. These drugs have, for the most part, been developed by drug manufacturers through their own research-and-development programs. Publicly supported medical research has also played a role, but even when basic breakthroughs occur in the laboratory of a university or other nonprofit institution, private industry is responsible for transforming the research discovery into a marketable product.

During the past decade the rate of introduction of new drugs has decreased appreciably. The average number of new chemical entities (i.e., truly new drugs) annually placed on the market since 1962 is roughly one-half the average for the preceding decade. According to Sam Peltzman, professor of economics at the University of Chicago, this decrease is attributable to the 1962 Kefauver-Harris Amendments to the Pure Food and Drug Act.[7] These amendments, which Congress passed in the emotional aftermath of the thalidomide tragedy, impose much more stringent requirements on drug companies for proof of efficacy and safety.

Drug manufacturers claim that, as a result, two to four additional years are now required to obtain the necessary approval for a new drug from the federal

Food and Drug Administration (FDA), with a considerable attendant increase in costs. Expenditures by drug manufacturers for research and development are now much greater than they were in the period when the number of new drug products was so much higher. Drug industry spokespersons contend that the delay in FDA approval places an even greater burden on them than the accompanying increase in costs by making it that much more difficult for manufacturers to anticipate the state of the market and technology. Peltzman further argues that the delay in the introduction of new drugs and the reduction in their number as a result of the more stringent FDA regulations is far more costly to the nation's health than the possible cost of some unsafe or inefficacious drug that might be marketed under less stringent legislation.[8]

The process of developing a new drug and bringing it on the market is indeed a long and expensive one. It may begin with (for example) the deliberate modification of a natural product that has a desired therapeutic effect, or with the accidental discovery that some compound acts in a desired way. Initial screening using rodents and other animals usually follows. Specialists in numerous disciplines, including biology, chemistry, and biochemistry, become involved at this stage. Developmental chemists undertake large-scale synthesis of the drug, and if continued testing reveals a significant therapeutic effect, toxicity studies are initiated. Usually dogs or monkeys are given the drug in the same way that it would be used with humans, and careful examinations are conducted to determine toxic effects.

If a compound gives promise of both efficacy and safety, at this point it is administered to humans under controlled conditions by physician investigators. If after extensive clinical trials the FDA approves the new drug application, the product can then be marketed.

Dr. Louis Lasagna, professor of pharmacology at the University of Rochester, has also commented on the inhibiting effects of the Kefauver-Harris Amendments. In addition, he speculates that perhaps "the fantastic output of the pharmaceutical industry (prior to 1962) preempted many additional contributions by tackling successfully the 'easier' development problems, and that post-'Golden Age' research is necessarily less productive because the nuts left to crack are the tougher ones."[9]

Comparing the dates of introduction of new drugs in the United States with dates for the same drugs in France, Germany, and England, Lasagna finds that for the period 1965–1969 the United States lagged an average of one year behind France, 1.6 years behind Germany, and 2.1 years behind England.[10] On the other hand, he notes that in the case of L-dopa, a spectacular new drug for the management of Parkinson's disease, FDA approval was obtained relatively swiftly. The drug was quickly placed on the market with the understanding that experience with it would be carefully assessed so that if unforeseen major problems arose, approval could be rescinded.

A 1971 FDA report contends that the number of new drugs representing "important therapeutic advances" has not been adversely affected by the 1962 amendments.[11] An extremely comprehensive comparison of new drugs in Great Britain and in the United States by Dr. William War-dell, however, reveals that since 1962 there has been "a substantial lag and a deficit ... in the introduction of new drugs to the American market."[12] Between 1962 and 1971, seventy-seven new drugs were introduced in Great Britain that were not available in the United States, while only twenty-one were available in the United States but not in Great Britain. Of eighty-two new drugs that became available in both countries, forty-three appeared first in Great Britain, with an average lead of 2.8 years, while twenty-five appeared first in the United States, with an average lead of 2.4 years. Fourteen were introduced in the same year in both countries.

Wardell identified several drugs that were available in Great Britain, but not in the United States, which British physicians considered of significant therapeutic value, including the use of salbutamol (albuterol) in asthma, the beta blocker in angina, co-trimoxazole in pyelonephritis, and carbenoxolene in gastric ulcer. A survey of American specialists revealed that very few of them were aware of the existence of these drugs, although those who were aware expressed a desire to have them available in the United States.[13] (The fact that so few American specialists knew of these drugs' existence — despite extensive discussion of them in professional journals — seems to testify to the importance of the detailer and drug industry advertising as sources of information on drugs for American physicians.)

The principal thrust of Wardell's and of Peltzman's work is that the present FDA regulations are heavily biased in the direction of keeping drugs off the market. This is done in the name of saving lives (by preventing unsafe drugs from reaching the market) and saving money (by preventing inefficacious drugs from reaching the market). The net result, however, may be unnecessary suffering or even loss of life because some drugs that would be efficacious for some patients are not available.

Wardell's analysis points to the fact that most adverse drug reactions in both Great Britain and the United States are associated not with the new or relatively untried drugs, but with drugs that have been long in use. He argues that paying more attention to postmarketing surveillance (which is much poorer in the United States than in many other countries) would do more to reduce drug hazards than the current American practice of relying on extensive animal testing and other premarketing screening procedures. The limitations of animal testing are highlighted by the fact that penicillin and fluroxene, two valuable drugs, are both lethal to some laboratory animals. Thus if these drugs were just being developed today, the clear evidence of their toxicity in animals would probably result in their rejection long before approval was sought to market them. On the other hand, it is not at all clear that present regulations would prevent a thalidomide from being marketed.[14]

Another crucial point underscored by both Lasagna and Wardell is that the availability of an efficacious drug for a particular condition is not sufficient reason to bar a less efficacious alternative from the market. Suppose, for example, that drug A is already on the market and is successful in the treatment of a disease 50 percent of the time, has no effect in 40 percent of cases, and is actually harmful in 10 percent. Further suppose that a new drug — drug B — is proposed for the same disease and that tests indicate it is effective only in 30 percent of cases and is harmful in 20 percent. Should approval to market drug B be withheld on the grounds that a more efficacious drug (drug A) is already available? Not necessarily. Drug B may actually be effective in a substantial number of cases where drug A is not; if so, to bar B from the market would be to deny a number of patients their only opportunity for effective therapy.

It is interesting to speculate what would happen if the regulatory standards that are applied to drugs in the United States were also applied to surgical procedures. Suppose no operation could be undertaken unless there was significant and conclusive evidence of both the efficacy and the safety of the procedure. Would tonsillectomies pass the test of efficacy? About a million are performed annually in the United States, yet many physicians are skeptical of their value except in special cases. Would surgery for lung cancer meet such a test? In Great Britain such surgery is undertaken much less often than in the United States. The ostensible reason these standards are not applied to surgery is that reliance is placed on the physician (and hospital) not to undertake or permit inappropriate procedures. Also, a patient who undergoes surgery that should not have been performed always has recourse to a malpractice suit (or at least the patient's family does).

Could the traditional approach to surgery be used with respect to prescription drugs? Under law a patient cannot obtain such drugs without a physician's prescription. No physician is under any compulsion to prescribe a drug unless one believes that its possible therapeutic benefits outweigh possible harm. Moreover, patients still have recourse to malpractice suits in cases of the physician's gross negligence.

The present approach of strict market controls on drugs really amounts to a vote of "no confidence" in physicians' ability to prescribe with judgment and care. If such a vote is warranted, it raises serious questions about the state of medical education, the organization of medical practice, and the usefulness of medical licensure.

A critical question for social choice in the drug field at this time is whether the United States should continue to place heavy emphasis on barring potentially unsafe drugs from the market at the cost of possibly delaying the introduction of helpful new drugs. A policy of extreme caution hardly seems warranted a priori since human lives are at stake either way the choice is made. If physicians are in fact ill equipped to function within a more permissive regulatory framework, perhaps the solution lies in the reform of medicine rather than in regulation of drugs.

Drugs and Ill Health

The overuse, abuse, and misuse of drugs constitute a major health problem in the United States. From the medical point of view, overuse occurs whenever a drug's net effect on health is harmful. Drug abuse is simply an extreme version of overuse, and usually refers to drug addiction. From the economic point of view, however, overuse must be defined differently. On the one hand, any drug use which did not yield a benefit equal to its cost would constitute economic overutilization, even if it were not detrimental to health. On the other hand, some use that *is* detrimental to health would not be characterized as overuse in economic terms if it increased satisfaction in other ways. Good health and long life are not the consumer's only goals.

From a health point of view one of the most overused drugs in the United States is alcohol. At least one of every twenty adults, and possibly as many as one in ten, consume alcohol at a level harmful to their health. Other drugs that are commonly overused include nicotine, caffeine, and aspirin. Prescription drugs that are believed to be objects of widespread overuse include tranquilizers, barbituates, and amphetamines. The abuse of heroin, cocaine, LSD, and other illegally obtained drugs is, of course, a major problem, but beyond the scope of this discussion.

What, if anything, should be done about the overuse of drugs? Education is one possible answer. If overuse is the result of ignorance, there is a clear and proper role for both private and public institutions in trying to help people make more intelligent use of their purchasing power. What about the adult who knows that drugs harm health but persists in drug overuse because it provides other satisfactions? Should such adults be free to make and carry out their own decisions regarding drug use? The answer to this, in my view, is that it depends on the nature and extent of the consequences of such use for others. For instance, overuse of alcohol, particularly outside one's home, may well imperil the comfort and safety of others, and in such a case government has the clear right to intervene. But the notion — so popular in some quarters — that government has the obligation and capacity to keep people from doing anything that seems foolish (even when there is no harm to others) should be firmly rejected by all who value a free society. In the case of health, the possibilities for intervention are almost without limit: one could first prohibit alcohol and then cigarettes, then try to curb overeating, then compel exercise, and so on.

That which government should refrain from compelling, however, the physician has every right and duty to try to accomplish by persuasion. The physician who is successful in persuading patients to reduce weight or eliminate cigarette smoking may be doing more for health than the one who has mastered the most esoteric diagnostic and therapeutic techniques.

A related problem concerning drugs is their misuse. It has been estimated that 1½ million persons are hospitalized each year as the result of adverse drug reactions. Many millions more experience adverse reactions not requiring hospitalization but producing considerable pain, discomfort, and disability.[15] Some "misuse" is inevitable so long as it is impossible to predict with certainty the way every patient will react to every drug. Other cases of misuse are clearly the fault of patients who fail (or refuse) to follow instructions. Much of the misuse, however, represents a failure of the medical care delivery system. Correction of such failure should be high on the agenda of health care educators and researchers. What is needed is more knowledge and more concern on the part of physicians and a closer articulation of the prescribing and dispensing functions. The current proliferation of specialization in medicine, for example, causes situations where a patient may be simultaneously taking several drugs prescribed by different physicians. The potential for harm, obviously great here, could be reduced if all the drugs were dispensed by a single knowledgeable pharmacist.

Drug Costs

Drug costs do not present as big a problem for social policy as do the effects of drugs on health. Drug expenditures account for about 10 percent of total health expenditures, and this share has tended to decline over time. The drug portion of the consumer price index has been relatively stable for many years, and has actually decreased during some. Even the average price of prescriptions, which was rising rapidly in the 1950s when new, expensive drugs were flooding the market, has been rising at only a moderate rate, and most of this change is due to an increase in the size of the average prescription.[16]

Although the problem of drug costs is not among the most pressing in the health field, several aspects are worthy of consideration. First, it should be noted that only a small part of the cost of drugs goes to pay for the materials and labor used to produce them. Of every dollar received by drug manufacturers, only about 40 cents is used for materials and supplies, production-worker wages, and other payroll. This is a smaller percentage than in almost any other industry, even including cosmetics.

Much of the drug sales dollar is used for marketing, including advertising. The exact percentage is not known, although Senator Gaylord Nelson (D.-Wisc.), a long-time critic of the drug industry, claims that it is as high as 25 percent of total sales — a much higher proportion than is spent by most manufacturing industries. The share of sales spent for research is more than 5 percent and less than 15 percent, but there is no agreement on the exact figure.

The rate of profit in drug manufacturing has been very high throughout the past quarter-century. In most years the drug industry has led all manufacturing in rate of return on stockholders' equity, and the rate has been one-and-one-half times the average of all industries combined. The reported rate is biased upward because the drug industry's heavy investment in research and development is not capitalized (as is investment in physical capital), but this accounting peculiarity would explain only a part of the "excess" profits. Other factors offered by the industry to explain its high rate of return, such as the high risk involved in marketing individual drug products or the need for research-and-development funds, are unconvincing. The major reasons for high profits are, rather, product differentiation and the absence of price competition among existing firms, aided by the role played by patents and exclusive process know-how in inhibiting competition from new firms.

There can be little doubt that drug prices could be reduced substantially if sharp cuts were made in advertising, research expenditures, and profits. Whether this would be desirable or not is another matter. It is naive to assume that the public interest always lies in the direction of lower prices. If lowering drug prices were to inhibit the development of useful new drugs, for instance, the public interest might be poorly served.

High profits have probably helped fuel the rapid expansion of the drug industry in the past. If there is less need for expansion now, profits could and probably should be lower. The charge that expenditures for drug marketing are excessive seems well supported, but these expenditures are likely to continue as long as they pay off for the manufacturers. Significant changes in drug marketing, therefore, are not likely to occur without significant changes in physicians' behavior.

One such change that has been urged on physicians is to prescribe "generically" whenever possible instead of specifying brand names. By prescribing generically the physician affords the pharmacist the option of filling the prescription with any manufacturer's version of that drug, including (presumably) the cheapest version. When a physician prescribes by *brand* name, the anti-substitution laws in most states forbid the pharmacist from substituting a generic equivalent. Those who defend brand-name prescribing, however — including, of course, brand-name drug manufacturers — maintain that generic prescribing would not result in significant savings for the patient. While acknowledging individual instances of huge price differences between the brand-name and generic versions of the same drug, they argue that there are so many drugs where the difference is small and so many where no generic version exists that total possible savings would be less than 10 percent.

Considerable controversy has arisen over whether generic drugs are in fact therapeutically equivalent to their brand-name counterparts. It has been shown, for example, that two manufacturers' versions of the same drug, although chemically equivalent, may not be therapeutically equivalent because of differences in rate of absorption within the body, among other reasons. Advocates of generic prescribing admit that not all chemically equivalent drugs dissolve at the same rate, but they question whether this is true for most drugs and they also note the lack of agreement among pharmacologists regarding therapeutically adequate rates of absorption and blood levels.

Yet another hot argument is now raging over whether pharmacists should be granted the right to substitute one manufacturer's version of a drug for another when the physician has prescribed a brand name. Those in favor of the right to substitute — including the American Pharmaceutical Association (a pharmacists' organization) — argue that if the pharmacist is aware of a cheaper alternative considered to be just as good, or better, than the brand name prescribed, the patient should be allowed this potential saving. Opponents of this right, however — including the Pharmaceutical Manufacturers Association (representing the drug industry) — argue that the physician knows the patient best and is in the best position to decide not only which drug but which brand of drug the patient should have.

A useful compromise position is the one adopted by the Kaiser Medical Group in California. On the bottom of their prescription blanks there is a little box and the notation, "Authorization is given for dispensing by nonproprietary name unless checked here." Thus if the physician wants to insure that the pharmacist dispenses the specific brand prescribed, the box is checked; if the physician does not mind a substitution being made, the box is left empty. The system, according to Kaiser officials, works quite well. It allows the physician to exercise strict control of treatment when considered necessary while permitting opportunities for savings in the cost of drugs in other cases.

The mere existence of alternatives, however, is no guarantee of savings. Lowering drug costs, it has been emphasized throughout, requires that physicians become more concerned with and knowledgeable about the drugs they prescribe. The prescription drug program of the Group Health Cooperative of Puget Sound in Washington State provides a good example of this. The cost per prescription in this prepaid plan — which covers hospitalization, physician's services, and out-of-hospital prescription drugs — is about one-half the national average. The principal reason for this is that the group's physicians have given a good deal of thought and attention to their prescribing. They will not prescribe a high-price brand-name drug if they know that an equally good lower-price version is available or that some cheaper drug product will do the same job. In addition, the group is able to buy drugs at more favorable rates because of its larger volume. Very little of the saving comes from greater technical efficiency in the running of the pharmacy; nearly all of it is in lower costs of the drugs purchased.

There are a substantial number of important drugs now available from only a single source whose patents will be expiring shortly. After the patents expire it is likely that these drugs will become available from several sources. The potential savings from generic prescribing or, what amounts to almost the same thing, from permitting pharmacists to practice brand substitution, will increase.

While many economists believe that drug prices are higher than they should be according to criteria of efficiency and equity, a few believe that even higher prices might be warranted as an inducement to develop and market drugs to treat relatively rare diseases. Some physicians have also expressed concern about the cost of developing drugs to treat rare diseases. If the potential market is small, and the cost of development high, it is clear that a profit-seeking firm will not undertake the required research. It has been proposed that some kind of subsidy is desirable to encourage such research. This argument runs counter to the economic point of view. Following that logic the state should subsidize guard rails on roads that are very seldom traveled (to prevent the "rare accident") and should spend money in many different ways that might conceivably result in saving a few lives.

Suppose those with the rare disease would be willing to pay a very large sum for an effective drug. At present, drug firms assume that even if their research produces an extremely valuable drug, they will not be able to charge anything close to its value to consumers. Fear of public opinion, government intervention, and the like preclude such a possibility. Because of this assumption potentially useful research and development, especially for rare diseases, may be shelved.

Ethical Problems

Significant ethical problems surround all aspects of medicine and several of the most troublesome ones involve drugs. Consider, for instance, the widespread use of placebos in medical practice. *Placebo* is the term applied to any harmless concoction (e.g., sugar and water) given to a patient under the pretense that it is an active drug. If the definition is broadly construed to include things like vitamins (when no vitamin deficiency is apparent), it appears that a significant proportion of all prescriptions are placebos. One British physician who kept a careful record of his prescriptions reported that 30 percent were in the placebo category.

Why do physicians prescribe placebos? To some extent because they constitute the safest therapy for treating hypochondria. By prescribing a placebo and thus pretending to acknowledge the seriousness of the patient's condition, the physician may be preventing that patient from resorting to harmful self-medication or to treatment from some unqualified or unscrupulous third party. Some physicians defend their practice of prescribing placebos by arguing that it "cements the physician-patient relationship": the patient who expects to be given a prescription may feel that the physician who fails to write one hasn't really done anything or doesn't really care to.

Cynics might say that physicians prescribe placebos in order not to lose customers; but the practice is also widespread in charity clinics and other settings where the question of patronage loss is less relevant.

Because of the strong psychological component in many illnesses, placebos often in fact work — i.e., have a favorable effect on health. On the other hand, they can of course be downright dangerous — by being totally useless — if prescribed after inadequate diagnosis or as a substitute for concentrated efforts to deal with serious problems.

The use of placebos undoubtedly adds to the public's expenditures for drugs, but it is not clear whether there is any less expensive way of dealing with the cases for which they are typically prescribed. Some might argue that if no prescription is indicated, the physician should take the time to explain the situation carefully to the patient in order to save the patient's money. But this may not be the most cost-effective way of dealing with the case; the physician's time also costs money — if not to the patient, then to the physician. Under fee-for-service where the patient pays for the drug separately, the physician's impulse is to write a prescription and get on to the next case without unnecessarily wasting time. Under a prepayment plan that covers the cost of prescriptions, the physician is more likely to weigh the cost of time against the cost of a placebo — ideally with the help of some organization formula.

Another ethical question is whether physicians should themselves dispense drugs for profit. One school of thought regards this as unethical, arguing that physicians would be tempted to overprescribe in order to increase their incomes. Exactly the same point, however, could be made concerning the tests and X rays that physicians recommend (and charge for), the surgery they perform, and the return visits they suggest. Indeed, if all drugs had to be administered by injection, this issue would not even arise. This is not to deny that abuses occur in the other areas just mentioned, but to say that the problem of insuring responsible physician behavior doesn't begin or end with the prescribing and dispensing of drugs. If a physician wants to take advantage of the patient's lack of medical knowledge, this can be done in many ways other than overprescribing.

The phenomenal rise in the importance of drugs during the past few decades, uncertainty concerning some of the basic facts about drug research, sales, and usage, and the limited amount of objective analysis of drug industry performance make it difficult to reach firm conclusions for social policy in this area. Whereas well-meaning critics of the drug industry continue to press for stricter government controls on drug development and marketing, other analysts are arguing that such controls seriously impede the war on disease. With respect to drug prices, my own view is that they are currently higher than they need be as a result of a wasteful distribution system and the lack of price competition within the industry. The crucial questions regarding drugs, however, relate not to cost but to the consequences of drugs on health. One weakness of the present system is the almost total absence of any connection between the retail sale of drugs and the practice of medicine. A related weakness is the limited knowledge many physicians have concerning drugs. Given the central role of the physician in medical care, it seems to me that the best way to achieve more rational prescribing and a more efficient, effective drug industry is by physicians becoming more knowledgeable about drugs. Education can help, but probably the strongest incentive, as in the case of hospital care, would be the inclusion of prescription drugs in prepaid capitation medical insurance plans so that the physician had a clear financial stake in the cost of drugs.

Supplementary Reading

Please see "Innovation and Shortage: The Yin and the Yang of the Health Sector" in Part 2.

CHAPTER 6

Paying for Medical Care

> Some saw health insurance primarily as an educational and public health measure, while others argued that it was an economic device to precipitate a needed reorganization of medical practice.... Some saw it as a device to save money for all concerned, while others felt sure that it would increase expenditures significantly.
>
> DANIEL S. HIRSCHFIELD,
> The *Lost Reform*, commenting on the campaign for compulsory health insurance in the United States at the time of World War I

How to pay for medical care? This question, which periodically has been the subject of vigorous debate in the United States for more than half a century, has moved to the forefront of public attention in the wake of rapid increases in the cost of care and heightened concern about inequality of access. More than a dozen different proposals for some type of national health insurance have been submitted in Congress, and major interest groups — private insurance companies, hospitals, organized medicine, and organized labor — have staked out their positions in great detail. Before considering the pros and cons of national health insurance and the implications of alternative proposals, a few general remarks about medical care finance and the present U.S. system are in order.

The most basic point, often obscured in public discussions, is that the public must pay for care under any system of finance. That is, the ultimate cost falls on families and individuals even when the payment mechanism makes it appear that the bills are being sent elsewhere. Except during an economic depression, no magic wand of finance can divert labor, capital, and other resources to medical care without resulting in a reduction in resources available for food, housing, education, recreation, or other goods and services. Nor is there any secret formula that can transfer the cost of health care to "government" or "business" without the burden eventually being borne by the public through more taxes, higher prices, or lower wages. Granted, the choice of financing system can make a significant difference to families at the highest and lowest levels of income, but the average family will have to pay the same share under any system.

Not that the method of financing medical care is irrelevant. On the contrary, the choice of financing system can have significant implications, especially for cost and access. This is particularly true when one considers that the financing system has two sides: how people pay for care and how providers are paid.

The two sides are sometimes linked in a single transaction, as in the traditional system when a patient buys services directly from a physician: the patient pays fee-for-service, and the physician is paid fee-for-service. Under the medical foundation system, however, as pioneered by the San Joaquin County Medical Society in California and now being copied in many other states, the patient (or the respective employer) pays an annual insurance premium, while the physician continues to be compensated on a fee-for-service basis. On the other hand, in the world-famous Mayo Clinic (and in several other large private group practices patterned after it), patients (or their insurance companies) pay fee-for-service, but the physicians receive a salary from the organization.

Besides fee-for-service, the principal ways in which consumers pay for medical care are either directly, through insurance premiums and taxes, or indirectly, through higher prices or lower wages if the taxes are levied on business firms. The principal ways of compensating physicians, aside from fee-for-service, are capitation (an annual fee for each person covered regardless of actual utilization of services), salary, or profit sharing (in group practices). Hospitals can be paid on the basis of their charges, retrospective costs, negotiated rates, or prospective budgets.

The Present System

The present system for financing medical care in the United States reflects the diversity and pluralism characteristic of American life in general. Unlike the small homogeneous democracies of Western Europe or the large centrally controlled nations such as the USSR and China, the United States has refrained from establishing a national medical care system just as it has refrained from a national system of education, police, and many other basic services. Of the more than $90 billion spent on health care in the United States in 1973, however, government was the source of about 40 percent, two-thirds of it federal monies and one-third from state and local governments. The next largest source was direct payment by patients, which amounted to about one-third of the total. Payments by private insurance companies (including Blue Cross, Blue Shield, and other nonprofit plans) amounted to about one-fifth, and the balance was supplied by philanthropy, company-operated health services, and miscellaneous other sources.

The relative importance of different financing sources varies greatly depending upon the type of expenditure. For instance, dental services, drugs, and eyeglasses, which together account for almost 20 percent of total expenditures, are paid for almost exclusively by patients, although there is a minor trend toward providing insurance coverage for these items.

Private insurance is most important in paying for hospital and physician costs. In general, the distribution between private insurance and direct patient payment tends to be influenced by the size of the expenditure and its variability. The more expensive the item and the more variable it is from family to family, the more likely it is that the insurance mechanism will be brought into play. Insurance is a method of avoiding risk, or, more accurately, of sharing risk. In some societies risk is shared through extended-family and kinship obligations, but organized insurance, either private or public, has become a major factor in the more impersonal, individualistic societies of the modern world.

Apart from the desire to share risk, many people seem to prefer the convenience of having medical care payments periodically deducted from their wages in the form of insurance premiums. The alternative would be voluntary saving in order to be able to pay for services when utilized. Even if the question of risk did not arise, that is, if a family knew for certain that its total medical expenditures would be $520 over the year, they might still prefer to have $10 per week deducted to cover the cost, rather than having to come up with the money at the time of treatment.

The government supplies most of the funds for public health programs (e.g., control of epidemics) and for medical research. This makes a great deal of economic sense inasmuch as these activities indirectly benefit large numbers of people. It would hardly be efficient to let individual consumer demand determine the size of public health or medical research programs. For instance, although basic scientific research on cancer stands to eventually benefit millions, which makes the *collective* demand for this research quite strong, the incentive for *individuals* to pay for cancer research is weak, since any future benefits will be made widely available regardless of who pays for the research now.

Whenever the action taken by an individual, household, or firm confers benefits (or imposes costs) on others and no feasible way exists of arranging direct compensation for these benefits (or costs), economists say there is an "externality." When externalities arise, there is an a priori case for some kind of governmental or collective action. For instance, if I am debating whether to be vaccinated for a contagious disease, my self-interest requires weighing the personal cost (time, money, side effects) against the personal benefit (immunity). Such a calculation ignores the external benefit, that is, the benefit to others, whose chances of getting the disease decrease as the number of immunized people increases. A calculation based on self-interest thus leads to an *undervaluation* of vaccination; hence economic efficiency requires that the decision not be left to a free market choice. Self-interest weighs private cost against private benefit; the optimum for society requires comparing social costs and social benefits. An example of an external cost is the pollution attributable to a factory smokestack. In choosing between a low-price dirty fuel and one that is cleaner but higher in price, the factory owner will probably ignore the pollution costs unless the government intervenes. The factory owner's private interest leads to choosing the "cheaper" fuel — even though the other fuel might really be cheaper if all costs (including pollution) are considered.

Most medical care does not involve externalities in the sense discussed above. The benefits of surgery, for instance, accrue primarily to the patient and the respective family. This is equally true of most medical interventions, with the notable exception of treatment of communicable diseases. Nevertheless, the share of government in paying for hospital care and physicians' services has grown rapidly in recent years for reasons that will be discussed below.

Before World War II the roles of both government and private insurance in health care were relatively much smaller than they are today; direct patient payment and philanthropy were relatively more important. Private insurance grew particularly rapidly in the 1940s and 1950s; in recent years its share of total expenditures has been fairly stable. Part of the original impetus for the private expansion of health insurance came from the health care providers, especially the hospitals, who were concerned about achieving certainty of payment and stability of revenue. Additional impetus stemmed from the increasing demand for medical insurance premiums as a fringe benefit in labor contracts. During World War II, for example, increases in fringe benefits were often exempt from federal ceilings on wages. And despite the lifting of wartime controls, the fact that employer contributions for medical insurance are not taxed as employee income continued to make this method of finance attractive to workers throughout the recent decades of high and rising personal taxes.

Another factor that has undoubtedly contributed to the growth of both private and public insurance is the increasing complexity of medical technology. Today it is possible and sometimes desirable to provide care at a level of expense far beyond the means of the average family except through the insurance mechanism.

The decline in the relative importance of voluntary philanthropy has been offset (some say more than offset) by "compulsory philanthropy" — i.e., by redistribution of income through government. This shift may reflect recognition that philanthropy frequently involves "external" benefits analogous to those discussed above. Suppose X is poor and sick and both A and B would like to see X better off. If A voluntarily gives X some money or arranges medical care for X, B will derive some pleasure from seeing the improvement in X without having spent a cent. If B is the one who makes the gift, A derives the same kind of benefit at no cost (to oneself). Under a system of voluntary philanthropy, neither A nor B is likely to give X as much as they would if full account were taken of their collective desire to see X better off. A good solution would be for A and B to get together and agree on a tax-supported program — that is, compulsory philanthropy. The undervaluation of philanthropy in the free market is thus similar to the undervaluation of vaccination previously discussed. The solution is also similar — some kind of government intervention to insure that the choices facing individuals reflect social costs and social benefits.

The rapid expansion of the government's share of health expenditures in recent years is probably due in part to an increase in egalitarian attitudes. It is not entirely clear, however, why there is apparently more support for redistributing income through subsidized medical care than for simply redistributing income directly and letting individuals decide how they want to spend their money. Where medical care for the poor involves using such groups for teaching and research purposes, as under much private philanthropy, significant external benefits probably accrue to those who are not poor. Many government-supported programs, however, are trying to eliminate these discriminatory practices.

Other motives may underlie changes in financing arrangements. For instance, some supporters of government health insurance predict that it will increase patients' bargaining strength *vis-à-vis* hospitals, physicians, and other providers, since a single large buyer (in this case, the government) is in a much better position to negotiate prices and supervise quality. It is also thought that national health insurance would provide the leverage to bring about needed changes in the organization and delivery of care. By changing the incentives facing the providers, the payment mechanism could be used to eliminate unnecessary hospitalization, to control drug prescribing, and to limit costs in general.

Sometimes the motivation for change is to improve the care process through integration of the payment and delivery systems, as in the Group Health Cooperative of Puget Sound (discussed in Chapter 5), which is a true consumers' cooperative. Patients own the hospital, engage the physicians, and serve as volunteers. Interestingly enough, where consumers have almost complete control, as in this system, they do not necessarily opt for maximum coverage: although the co-op has a very comprehensive plan, it has refused to cover abortion services or out-patient tranquilizing drugs.

Although motives are diverse, support for a change in medical care finance is widespread. Republicans and Democrats, liberals and conservatives, the AMA and the AFL-CIO all agree that *some* kind of national health insurance is desirable. Underlying this consensus, however, are sharp disagreements concerning *who* should be covered, *what* kind of coverage should be provided, and *how* the plan should be financed, administered, and implemented.

Who?

The debate over *who* should be covered boils down to determining whether there should be universal coverage or whether federal payment for insurance should be limited to families and individuals with low income.

Those who favor the latter approach argue that the primary objective of a national health insurance program should be to remove the financial barrier to care for the poor. Since the average family has to pay for care one way or another, it is argued, the simplest solution is to let everyone but the poor buy their own insurance, perhaps with the encouragement of tax deductions for premiums paid. Expenditures for medical care, it has been noted, account for a significant proportion of national income. Why, it is asked, should many additional tens of billions of dollars be brought into the federal budget only to be dispersed again in local communities to pay for the care of individuals who could have financed that care through nongovernmental mechanisms? Some observers further contend that a system of universal insurance would put an unnecessary burden on the federal fiscal system and possibly endanger other important government programs.

Arguments made in support of universal coverage take many forms. One is that access to medical care should be a matter of right, just as police and fire protection and other essential services are provided by the government to all citizens regardless of income. A particularly strong case is made for providing children with access to care regardless of whether their parents can afford it or have made provision for it. Access for children is held to be an essential ingredient in the American commitment to equality of opportunity, and a comparison is drawn between medical care and schooling. The analogy is not perfect, however: free public education is often justified partially in terms of significant externalities, which is more difficult to establish with regard to many types of medical care.

Coupled with the philosophical argument that medical care is everyone's "right" is a practical argument that cautions against making too many benefits conditional on low income. If the price one pays for medical care, housing, children's college education, child care, and other goods and services depends on having a low income, there will be less incentive for individuals to try to raise their incomes.

Universal compulsory coverage is also advocated as the only effective way to deal with the problem of the "free rider." There are many people, it is argued, who can afford to buy health insurance but don't. If they or their dependents become seriously ill and incur huge bills, the community feels obliged to provide care. These people are in effect "free riders" on the rest of the community.

One telling argument in favor of universal coverage is that the level of benefits and the quality of administration would have to be high enough to satisfy the majority of Americans, whereas a special plan for the poor might quickly degenerate to a second-class level. True, theoretically the best way to help the poor is to redistribute income, but it might be more feasible politically to achieve some redistribution with a national health insurance plan.

This seems to be the case in Great Britain, where the National Health Service (NHS) makes care available to all segments of the population. There are admittedly regional differences in quantity and quality of facilities, and the ability to use the system effectively tends to vary with social class. On balance, however, the NHS is regarded as having introduced a significant element of equality and justice into British life, and it commands wide public approval on that account.

What?

The debate over *what* should be covered by a U.S. national health insurance plan takes many forms, including quibbles over such details as cosmetic surgery and types of eyeglasses. The most basic cleavage, however, is between those who favor insurance only for "catastrophic" costs (major-risk insurance) and those who favor comprehensive "first-dollar" coverage. One argument for limiting insurance to catastrophic costs proceeds from fairly orthodox principles of public finance. Several leading health economists, including Martin Feldstein of Harvard, have been among the leading proponents of major-risk insurance. The essential point is that insurance lowers the net price to the consumer and therefore encourages one to buy more care than if one had to pay the whole cost out of pocket. Feldstein argues that the more comprehensive the coverage, the greater the "welfare loss" entailed in society collectively "overconsuming" medical care at the expense of other goods and services which, at the margin, they value more highly.[1]

It is the "restaurant check" problem, writ large. When a group goes to a restaurant and decides to split the bill evenly, there is a tendency for individuals to spend more than they would if each paid for one's own order. In Feldstein's terms, there is a "welfare loss" from check splitting; nevertheless, the practice is widespread, and not without reason. One advantage is the reduced cost of "administration" — figuring out who ordered what and how much each owes. A second reason is that to the extent that a group meal is a social event, a party where each person is both host and guest, check splitting is conducive to the group feeling. These observations have some relevance to the question of medical insurance as well.

The catastrophic or major-risk approach has a great deal of political appeal because the premiums would be very much lower than for comprehensive plans, but a number of questions and objections may be raised concerning it. First, since initial expenditures would be paid by the patient and only large subsequent expenditures by insurance, there would be less incentive for persons to seek early care or preventive treatment; rather, the emphasis would be on expensive tertiary care. Second, the catastrophic approach would impose a large administrative burden on both patients and the government. Every family would have to maintain comprehensive records on all medical care expenditures in anticipation of eventually exceeding the deductible amount and becoming eligible for insurance coverage, and the government would have to establish means for checking these records. Most proposals call for the deductible to vary with the level of income of the family, so additional checking would be required to determine each family's income level in relation to its medical expenditures. The incentive to try to lump expenditures into the year when the deductible is exceeded, as well as the temptation to indulge in more flagrant forms of chicanery, would be very great.

Major-risk insurance would not deter utilization once the deductible had been satisfied, but it is the marginal expenditure over which the patient frequently has the most discretion. In hospital care, for example, the marginal decision frequently is whether to remain an extra day or so. The first several days' stay is often determined primarily by medical considerations; the last day or two are usually much more likely to be subject to patient preference. Given the size of the deductibles now proposed for major-risk insurance (about 10 percent of income, with an upper limit of about a thousand dollars), the average hospitalized patient would satisfy the deductible in the first several days and thereafter be under little or no financial pressure to cut short one's stay.

Moreover, it is not clear how the provision of major-risk insurance by the federal government would prevent families from also acquiring "first-dollar" or "shallow" coverage from private insurance companies if they so desired. It should be noted that although major-risk insurance in various forms is now available from private insurance companies, the demand for it is less that overwhelming. If major-risk insurance is really what people desire in the way of medical care coverage, why don't they buy it now? And why do union leaders and representatives of other groups seek more coverage? I believe one reason is because people want an easy, convenient, systematic way of *paying* for medical care. It is a great mistake to view the purchase of health insurance as simply the result of the desire to avoid risk.

Finally, it should be noted that the major-risk approach concentrates exclusively on the patient and does nothing about organization of care, problems of access, or efficiency of delivery systems. In my view, its appeal is extremely deceptive. It seems like a cheap way of getting out of a crisis, but it offers little hope of solving the major health care problems now facing the American public.

How?

The disagreements over the *how* of national health insurance fall into three main categories: how to raise money; how to administer the plan or plans; and how (or whether) to use the financing system to change the organization and delivery of care.

Governments raise money through taxes. The principal taxes being proposed for national health insurance — indeed, the only ones likely to yield sufficient revenue — are the income tax and the payroll tax. The former is believed to be more progressive (that is, taking a greater proportion of income as income rises) and thus likely to result in more redistribution to the poor. Professor Mark Pauly of Northwestern University points out, however, that while this is certainly true of an ideal income tax, the existing system is "shot through with exclusions, deductions and special categories of income," and that the higher income tax rates required for national health insurance may cause more distortion.[2]

Much time and effort have been spent debating whether an increased payroll tax should be paid by the employer or the employee or both. This is largely a spurious issue because the ultimate burden would be borne by the public in the form of either lower wages or higher prices. As Pauly notes, "The 'employers share' is really a piece of political jim-crackery, designed to get the people, most of whom are employees, to agree to levy a higher tax on themselves than they would if the true tax burden were made clear."[3]

A question related to the choice of tax is whether expenditures and tax receipts should be linked through a medical insurance trust fund or whether the level of expenditures should be set independently and financed from the government's general revenue. Under a payroll tax trust fund arrangement, the size of the program would be affected by fluctuations in business conditions. Some people believe that it would be desirable to have benefits closely related to costs, while others prefer to have the benefit level set independently of the government's revenue position. The two groups apparently agree that closely gearing benefits to tax receipts would make the government more reluctant to raise benefit levels, but they differ over whether this restraint would be desirable.

One of the bloodiest battles over national health insurance concerns the manner in which the plan or plans should be administered. At one extreme is the proposal for a single insurance fund administered by the government. At the other extreme is the argument that universal coverage could be achieved by requiring every individual (or the respective employer) to obtain coverage from a private insurance company, with the government's role limited to setting minimum standards and paying premiums for the poor. Not surprisingly, the private insurance companies regard any proposals for a single government-managed fund as a threat to their very survival. They have consequently been fighting tenaciously in an effort to reserve an important role for themselves in whatever system is finally adopted, an effort which most knowledgeable political observers believe will succeed.

Advocates of a single government plan are fond of pointing out the efficiency with which the old age and survivors program is administered by the federal government. The analogy, however, is imperfect. Social Security payments are relatively simple to administer; the provision of medical services or reimbursement for same is a much more complex task, as shown by the problems of payment delay and overpayment encountered with Medicare and Medicaid. Some degree of pluralism and competition in the administration of national health insurance is in my view desirable, if only because it would allow for more flexibility and innovation than is likely to be forthcoming from a single government agency.

One beneficial consequence of a single plan, however, is that it would facilitate control of total health expenditures. This has been demonstrated in England, which has a single national plan and devotes a much smaller proportion of its gross national product to health care than does the United States. Indeed, close control of expenditures and the greater equality mentioned previously seem to be the principal benefits of Britain's National Health Service. The expectation that it would emphasize preventive and early care, or that it would encourage great efficiencies in the production of medical care, do not, in the main, seem to have been realized.

The final point of major disagreement is over whether any new financing system should be used to change the organization and delivery of care. Present-day organized medicine is, on the whole, opposed to any changes in the traditional system; most physicians would like to see any national financing system limited to the payment of bills. The opposing view is that unless national insurance is used to modify current practices, costs will skyrocket and possibly destroy the system — a compelling argument, especially in view of the experience of Medicare and Medicaid. Thus if national health insurance is to be successful in improving access to services for the poor without resulting in a diminution in needed services for everyone else, then the financing system will have to put pressure on the delivery system to eliminate waste and inefficiency or else face ruinous inflation.

HMOs

National health insurance proposals that seek to use the financing mechanism to change the organization of medical care rely heavily on the creation and encouragement of health maintenance organizations (HMOs). Dr. Paul Elwood, one of the most active proponents of this concept, describes an HMO as "an organization which provides comprehensive medical care, including preventive, diagnostic, outpatient, and hospital services, to a voluntarily enrolled consumer population in return for a fixed, prepaid amount of money."[4] The key elements are comprehensive coverage, prepayment, and an organization that takes responsibility for availability and quality of services.

Two principal types of HMOs are already in operation. One is the prepaid group-practice plan as developed by Kaiser, the Group Health Cooperative of Puget Sound, and a few other organizations; the other is the medical care foundation as developed by the San Joaquin County Medical Society. In the former type, there is only one insuring agency, the physicians are either salaried or share the income of the group partnership, and the hospitals are usually owned and managed by the plan. The foundation approach is more varied, typically involving many insurance companies, physicians compensated by fee-for-service, and independent hospitals. The foundation is considered an HMO, however, for it undertakes to monitor the utilization and charges of the individual physicians and guarantees to third-party payers that annual per capita costs will not exceed a specified amount. The foundation approach is less organized in the sense that patients can seek care from any physician who is part of the plan. Also, physicians may practice either alone or in groups, and are free to work as much or as little as they wish.

Many advantages are claimed for HMOs. First, membership in an HMO implies more than simply having health insurance (which has been likened to having a "shopping license"), because the organization undertakes the responsibility of providing care — i.e., it guarantees *access*. According to the late Ray Brown, a health care expert, "The greatest worry and frustration of the American public with the health care system does not have to do with cost, but rather has to do with the public's feeling that it is medically disengaged. ... By having a single and known organization responsible for a particular set of individuals, those individuals are by this means wired or plugged into the health care system; that is, they know where they are supposed to go, and they know who is responsible to do something about it when they get there."[5]

Because the HMO provides *comprehensive* coverage, it alters incentives for the patient. In particular, patients are less likely to seek hospitalization for diagnostic work and other care that could be provided on an ambulatory basis than under health insurance plans where coverage is limited to care provided in the hospital. The HMO also alters incentives for physicians whose income is determined by annual capitation payments and who are consequently less likely to provide or order unnecessary care as a way of increasing their incomes. True, the temptation still exists in the foundation HMO, where physicians are paid fee-for-service, but the foundation acts as a counterweight through education, persuasion, and threats to withhold payment.

One advantage to providers in prepaid group practices is that they know approximately what their income will be and what services they will be called upon to provide, making it much easier to plan budgets and workforce requirements. Some HMO enthusiasts even maintain that health levels will be raised because providers will be more strongly motivated to keep patients healthy (in order to minimize the use of services).

Opponents of the HMO concept are both skeptical of its supposed advantages and critical of what they consider its drawbacks. Some health economists, for example, doubt whether there are significant economies of scale to be realized in large groups of physicians. Other health experts question whether physicians can do much to maintain the health of their patients even given the incentives to do so. A few critics have even questioned whether HMOs really lower hospitalization rates.

One specific disadvantage of HMOs, it is argued, is that providers will skimp on patient care because their income is unaffected by the amount of care delivered. Indeed, in some HMOs the physician's income is *increased* if there is less hospitalization or few prescriptions. Furthermore, the concern has been expressed that HMOs will try to enroll only the best risks. It is alleged that even if they do a wonderful job for their members, they will not serve the total community, and they will tend to throw the greatest burdens on other providers.

What does experience with existing HMOs suggest about these claims and counterclaims? With respect to hospital utilization the evidence is reasonably clear-cut: hospitalization (measured in patient-days) is lower for those covered by HMOs than for comparable populations covered by conventional insurance. The savings involved are at least 15 percent and may be as high as 30 percent. Moreover, these savings do not seem to be offset by higher out-of-hospital utilization. The savings are more dependable for prepaid group-practice plans than for foundations, although the San Joaquin Foundation, the oldest and best-established one, has an excellent record.

There is still considerable controversy, however, concerning *how* HMOs reduce hospitalization. Is it because physicians stand to benefit from lower hospitalization? Is it because patients have equally good coverage for ambulatory care? Health economist Herbert Klarman has suggested that control of bed supply may be the critical variable. If beds are not available, they can't be used. Just restricting the bed supply may not be enough to lower hospital utilization over the long run, however. If physicians and patients regard the supply as unduly restrictive, they will press for expansion or drop out of the plan. What is needed, apparently, is fewer beds plus an "approach" to medical practice that makes the smaller supply tolerable. This "approach" encompasses the incentives and constraints facing the physician, the training and professional "socialization," and a feeling on the part of the patient that one's needs are being met.

The skepticism about HMOs improving the health of their members seems to be justified. Apart from some old studies of infant mortality in HIP (Health Insurance Plan of Greater New York), no major health effects of HMOs have been reported. Indeed, it is significant that none of the best-known HMOs make any important claims with respect to health. This is consistent with my view that health differences are determined largely by genetic factors, environment, and life-style. It is unlikely that variations in the quantity, quality, or organization of medical care can make a significant difference for the health of populations as a whole, although obviously the impact in individual cases can be very great.

If there is little evidence that HMOs improve health, there is even less evidence that HMO physicians tend to neglect the legitimate health needs of their patients. Indeed, so long as enrollment in a HMO is voluntary and alternative modes of care are available, the HMO must satisfy its customers or lose them.

On balance, then, existing HMOs have demonstrated that it is possible to control cost without jeopardizing patient health. When a group of physicians sets out to eliminate unnecessary utilization and curb wasteful practices, great savings are possible, particularly regarding hospitalization and drugs. Many physicians are resisting changes in the way they are paid, but unless the financing system is used to modify the behavior of physicians and hospitals, a national health insurance plan might do more harm than good. Forward-looking physicians might well consider August Heckscher's observation: "The prevailing structure of medical care — the doctor in solo practice dealing on a fee-for-service basis with the individual patient — is not part of the eternal order of things. It is a social convention, and like all social conventions, it is subject to reexamination, to development, to change."[6]

Concluding Comments

More than fifty years ago, at the time of World War I, there was a strong movement for compulsory health insurance in the United States. Its advocates, however, were divided (as are present advocates of national health insurance) over its ultimate purpose. Some wanted to control costs, others to improve health, and still others to make access more equal. In contrast to the present situation, significant opposition to compulsory health insurance came from many important labor leaders (including Samuel Gompers, then head of the American Federation of Labor), who opposed social insurance as "paternalistic." The medical profession, originally in favor of the proposal, gradually became a significant source of opposition, partly in response to the influence of the commercial insurance companies.

According to Daniel S. Hirschfield, the fundamental reason for the original failure of compulsory health insurance was that its major proponents were reformers who argued that traditional personal liberty and individual responsibility had to give way to new social and economic conditions — a position that the great majority, the public, did not share.[7]

At present, according to journalist Jonathan Spivak, "rising costs are the forcing factor for political action." I think he is correct, but I am not so sure of the corollary he adds — namely, that "cost considerations will also dominate the changes in the delivery system."[8] A serious attempt to deal with the cost problem — say, by moving to a capitation system of payment (including hospitalization, tests, and drugs) — is likely to run into opposition from physicians, drug companies, and possibly the insurance companies. Because the groups that think they have a great deal to lose will fight tenaciously, the most likely result will be a compromise that protects their interests. If the past is a good guide to the future, the emphasis is likely to shift to getting legislation that *appears* to serve great and noble purposes. Then, if the system in fact fails to live up to the expectations, the failure can be blamed on the administrators or on subsequent Congresses for failing to pass sufficient funds, or on the health professionals for sabotaging the programs.

Significant compromises are likely in order to overcome the objections of specific interest groups. Such compromises will probably tend to increase spending, while leaving organization and delivery unchanged. The only hopeful possibility is that representatives of other organized groups, such as business and union leaders — who in a sense represent workers, consumers, and taxpayers — will insist on changes that really make a difference. The time is past for either superficial measures or just pouring more money into the present system.

I am not so naive as to think we can or should develop a system of paying for medical care incongruent with the approach to other major problems in our society. The degree of equality, the nature of incentives and constraints, and the character and extent of government intervention must bear some relationship to arrangements in other sectors. The significance and economic importance of health care, however, are now so great that decisions taken with respect to this sector can substantially influence other areas. A responsible and effective policy for health and medical care, therefore, could become a cutting edge to help reshape our approach to other social problems.

Supplementary Reading

Please see "We Can't Have Everything: The Role of Payments for Volume and Choice of Provider in Fueling Health Expenditures" in Part 2.

CONCLUSION

Health and Social Choice

> The organization of medicine is not a thing apart which can be subjected to study in isolation. It is an aspect of culture whose arrangements are inseparable from the general organization of society.
>
> WALTON H. HAMILTON
> Medical Care for the
> American People

In the preceding chapters, I have discussed the major problems of health and medical care now facing the American people and have delineated the different social choices that must be made. These problems — high cost, inadequate access, and unsatisfactory health levels — have been examined from the economic point of view, which stresses the need to allocate scarce resources efficiently in order to best satisfy diverse human wants. For most Americans, better health is not the only, or even the most important, goal. For most Americans, more medical care is not the only, or even the most promising, route to better health.

The approach of this book has been to explore the relationship between health and such socioeconomic factors as income, education, and lifestyle and to examine in detail the principal elements of medical care: the physician, the hospital, and drugs. Economic analyses of these elements reveal significant opportunities for reorganizing care in order to moderate costs and improve access. In particular, Chapter 6 (on paying for medical care) indicated the central role of the financing system in this process.

Review

In this chapter, I shall summarize my policy recommendations, but before doing so it will be useful to restate here some of the principal conclusions about health and medical care that form the basis for the recommendations. One such conclusion is that health status (as measured by mortality, morbidity, or other indexes) depends on many things besides medical care. For most of human history, people's health has depended on their economic well-being (their real income). Adequate food supply, clean water, protection from the elements — these are historically critical factors affecting life expectancy and the avoidance of disability. In modern developed countries, income no longer seems to be a significant determinant of health except for the very poor, and particularly with regard to infant mortality (although even here differences in income have less effect than formerly).

Current variations in health among individuals and groups are determined largely by genetic factors, environment, and life-style (including diet, smoking, stability of family life, and similar variables). To be sure, changes in the health of the population over time are influenced by medical care — but mainly through scientific advances, not through changes in the quantity of care. The most rapid of these gains occurred between 1930 and 1955, largely due to the development of relatively inexpensive, highly effective drugs for the prevention or treatment of influenza and pneumonia, tuberculosis, and other infectious diseases. The current major health problems — heart disease, cancer, accidents, emotional illness, and viral infections — are more difficult to solve with the available medical technology.

In developed countries the marginal contribution of medical care to life expectancy is very small. That is, variations in mortality across and within countries do not seem to be related to differences in the availability of physicians or other medical care inputs. Medical care, however, performs other functions besides reducing mortality and morbidity. Particularly important are the caring function (sympathy, reassurance, relief of anxiety) and the validation function (provision of professional information about health status). Moreover, some of the high cost of medical care, especially in hospitals, is for amenities consistent with the general level of affluence in our society. People who live comfortably when they are well expect to do the same when they are sick.

Another aspect of medical care that preceding chapters have underlined is the overwhelming importance of the physician as principal decision maker. Even though only 20 percent of health care expenditures are for physicians' services and less than 10 percent of all health care workers are physicians, it is the physician who determines most of what happens in the health care process. The physician's role is particularly important with respect to the *cost* of care, because physicians usually make the pivotal decisions concerning hospitalization, surgery, tests, and drugs. Given the uncertainties about the effect of medical care on health, there is frequently a wide range of choice open to the physician on these matters. It follows that a concern with cost requires concentrating on the physician — particularly the criteria for admission to medical school, the nature of the physician's education and training, and, most important, the incentives and constraints faced once set up in practice.

The physician is also important with regard to the problem of access, although the common notion that simply increasing the number of physicians will provide a quick and easy solution is a mistaken one. The general problem of access to medical care is mainly a question of access to primary care and to emergency care. It is furthermore a question of finding a physician or an organization to take complete, continuing responsibility for all of a family's health needs. The problem arises principally from the growth of specialty and subspecialty medicine, not from an overall shortage of physicians. The general solution does not lie in increasing the number of such specialists, but in reorganizing the delivery system to make greater use of nurse clinicians and other physician extenders working under the supervision of physicians.

While the physician's behavior is of critical importance, the hospital is where the most money is spent and where costs have been rising most rapidly. Thus the hospital is where the greatest potential exists for stemming the increase in medical care costs. Moderating hospital costs can be accomplished primarily by moderating utilization — that is, by eliminating unnecessary admissions and reducing unduly long stays. Additional savings could be achieved by closing inefficient hospitals — thus bringing about higher occupancy rates — and by establishing better coordination among the remaining institutions. It is particularly important right now to stop subsidizing the creation of new hospital capacity, which at present is creating excess capacity and consequently inappropriate utilization.

Whereas cost considerations are central to the hospital problem, drugs are important primarily because of their tremendous potential to affect health for good or for harm. Most of the major advances in health over the past forty years are traceable to the introduction of new drugs. Inappropriate use of drugs (to say nothing of drug abuse), on the other hand, is now a significant source of ill health. For most people, drugs are only secondarily an economic or cost problem; drug expenditures and prices have not been rising at an unduly rapid rate in recent years. The sharp decrease in the number of new drugs coming onto the American market since the Kefauver-Harris Amendments of 1962, however, may indicate that this country is putting too much emphasis on premarketing controls and not enough on postmarketing surveillance.

Although the cost of drugs is not a crucial problem, significant opportunities for savings nevertheless exist. In the main, it is up to the physicians to take advantage of these opportunities, which they are most likely to do if they are given a financial stake in the cost of drugs. With respect to both drugs and hospitals, it has been shown that physicians can reduce costs without harming their patients' health, although they have little incentive to do so under the conventional fee-for-service payment system. When payment is made on an annual capitation basis that includes hospitalization, tests, and drugs, physicians are motivated to examine more closely the way they practice. Inasmuch as the financing of medical care, its organization, and its delivery are closely interrelated areas, it is naïve to think that solutions can be found in one without considering the others.

The Limits of Economics

One of the principal objectives of this book has been to show how the economic point of view can help us understand health problems. It is not my intention, however, to suggest that economics provides easy and ready solutions to the basic social problems that underlie questions of health and medical care. On the contrary, there are important limitations to economics.

One kind of limit is set by what economics can contribute *now*; that is, there are deficiencies in our theoretical framework and in our empirical knowledge that currently prevent us from answering particular questions about the health field. For instance, available economic theory is weak in explaining the behavior of nonprofit institutions and professional organizations, both of which are so important in medical care. Application of the traditional "theory of the firm," which assumes that organizations producing goods and services try to maximize profits, can yield many useful predictions regarding business decisions about prices, wages, composition and rates of output, and so on. In a voluntary nonprofit hospital, however, such decisions are usually the result of a "tug-of-war" among hospital administrators, the medical board, trustees, and the house staff. Furthermore, the motives of each of these groups differ, and their relative strengths vary, from hospital to hospital. Thus additional "theories of the firm" are needed to reflect the complexities.

Another troublesome aspect of economic theory is the assumption of perfect information. The elementary competitive model assumes that patients, physicians, and other decision makers possess all the necessary relevant information — about prices, production possibilities, usefulness of various therapies, and so on. In the real world, of course, such information may be difficult or even impossible to obtain. High information costs are characteristic of many health care markets; frequently the only way a person can know whether one needs to see a physician is to see a physician. At present most economic research on information costs and search is purely theoretical, but some day it may yield fruitful empirical insights into the behavior of patients and physicians.

Still another area of behavior that has important implications for health involves what goes on within the family. Whereas economists frequently treat the family (or household) as a basic unit of analysis and then seek to explain its behavior *vis-à-vis* the rest of the world, there has been relatively little effort so far to explain behavior *within* the household. The importance of the concept of investment in human capital is now recognized, however, and we know that much of this investment takes place within the family in the form of preschool learning and health care.

The consequences of intrafamily behavior for matters of health and general welfare can thus be significant. To take an intractable health problem of increasing concern as an example: Why do some parents go to extraordinary lengths to maintain and improve their children's health, while others are neglectful and still others even abuse and maim their children? These are difficult subjects to study empirically, however, because they involve no formal markets, no exchange of money, nor even the kind of input data available for studies of schooling or medical care.

In addition to theoretical weaknesses, there are serious limits to economists' current ability to estimate quantitative relationships between variables, even where theory predicts the direction of effects. For instance, economics can be used to predict that a decrease in the price of medical care will result in *some* increase in the amount of care demanded, but an effective policy decision would require an accurate estimate of the *degree* of response (termed "elasticity"). A consensus regarding the probable range of demand and supply elasticities in medical care markets is emerging only slowly. Similarly, we need better estimates of how cost is related to scale of production in medical care before making definitive judgments about the advantages or disadvantages of encouraging group practice or other changes in organization. Furthermore, every so often these relationships must be reestimated because, unlike relationships studied by natural scientists, economic relationships can and do change over time. Thus one of the limits of economics is that we must periodically discover anew the quantitative answers to old questions.

To keep these limitations in proper perspective, it should be noted that health economics is a relatively new field. The first national conference on the subject was held in 1962, the first international conference in 1973. There are perhaps only a hundred economists in the United States who devote all or most of their time to problems of health and medical care; by contrast, there are five times as many agricultural economists even though health care accounts for a much larger share of the gross national product than does agriculture. Nevertheless, the field has made considerable progress in the past decade, and the deficiencies mentioned above are, in principle at least, remediable. New theoretical insights, better data, and more sophisticated analyses will no doubt cause present limits to recede.

There are, however, other limits of an even more fundamental nature. At the root of most of our major health problems are *value choices*: What kind of people are we? What kind of life do we want to lead? What kind of a society do we want to build for our children and grandchildren? How much weight do we want to give to individual freedom? how much to equality? how much to material progress? how much to the realm of spirit? How important is our own health to us? How important is our neighbors' health to us? The answers we give to these questions, as well as the guidance we get from economics, will and should shape health care policy.

My own view is that we must quickly come to grips with the tremendous inequality in our nation. Imagine how critical we would be of a family which permitted some of its members to live in great luxury while other members lacked a minimum of basic goods and services. At the community level this is precisely the condition we tolerate. It is only a short walk from the opulence of upper Park Avenue to the rat-bitten, lead-poisoned children of East Harlem, but for our institutions that distance represents a chasm they seem powerless to bridge. Not that New York City is the only or the worst offender. The gap between the oil barons of Texas and the state's Chicano migrant farm workers is as large as any that can be found in New York. Paradoxically, the survival of our treasured personal freedom and independence may depend on our explicitly acknowledging a decent amount of interdependence and responsibility for one another.

The problem of inequality should be faced head on — in ways that do least damage to the efficient performance of the economy. Too often a concern for the poor has been used to justify minimum wages, price regulations, rent controls, and other devices that interfere with the competitive price system. This system (as Soviet planners have discovered) provides the most efficient mechanism for allocating scarce resources, even though it may result in a distribution of income which is socially and morally unacceptable.

While elementary justice seems to require greater equality in the distribution of medical care, the question is complicated by the fact that the poor suffer deprivation in many directions. Economic theory suggests it might be better to redistribute income and allow the poor to decide which additional goods and services they want to buy. As a practical matter, however, it may be easier to achieve greater equality through a redistribution of services (such as medical care) than through a redistribution of money income.

Recommendations

The recommendations that follow are based not only on my understanding of the economics of health and medical care, but also on my value judgments regarding what constitutes responsible policy in this field. As economist John Maurice Clark once wrote, "There are two worlds, the world of impersonal investigation of cause and effect, and the world of desires, ideals and value judgments. The natural sciences deal with the first, ethics with the second. . . . The peculiarity of economics is that it is called upon to bridge this gap."[1]

These are my principal policy recommendations:

1. *Universal comprehensive insurance.* Universal health insurance that meets nationally established minimum standards of benefits, with periodic upward readjustment of the minimum as technology changes and per capita income rises, should be established by Congress. The program should be universal because the best way of meeting the nation's responsibility to the poor is by integrating them into the same system covering the great mass of society. Another reason is that when care is provided only to those receiving less than a specified income, benefits are very difficult to administer and the system generates antisocial incentives. Participation should be compulsory to overcome the "free rider" problem and to improve the equality of opportunity for children.

A national health insurance plan to which all (or nearly all) Americans belonged could have considerable symbolic value as one step in an effort to forge a link between classes, regions, races, and age groups. It will be more likely to serve that function well if not too much is expected of it — if it is not oversold — particularly with respect to its probable impact on health. If too much is promised, then instead of being of positive symbolic value it may serve as another source of divisiveness. For each group may become convinced that they alone are being cheated, that the promised benefits are being realized by others but not by them.

2. *Decentralized delivery systems.* Most health services should be produced and delivered locally. While there are very few advantages in centralized control of delivery, there are many disadvantages, including a greater likelihood of high costs, bureaucratic rigidity, low morale among providers, and an inability to meet the diversity of local needs. A few, less frequently used, tertiary services should not be provided locally but at regional medical centers.

3. *Capitation payments for enrolled populations.* Capitation payment that covers hospitalization, medical care, and drugs has proven in practice to be convenient for the patient and easy to administer; most important of all, it leads to significant reductions in cost without jeopardizing health. Moreover, within a capitation system individual providers can be compensated in a variety of ways.

4. *Competition* (wherever possible) *among alternative health plans.* Although coverage should be compulsory, choice of plan should be voluntary. The economies of scale in medical care are not so great as to justify the creation of huge, monopolistic organizations. Except in areas of low population density, it would be more efficient to have most services (primary and secondary care) provided by several organizations in order to benefit from competitive pressures and to increase the range of choices available to consumers and providers.

5. *Elimination of many of the restrictions on use of health workforce experimentation with institutional licensure; and greater use of "physician extenders."* Improved access requires round-the-clock availability, an organization that takes continuing responsibility for its patients, and a good fit between the needs of the

patient and the skills and training of the provider. There is a continuum of health needs, and there should be a continuum of health care personnel to meet those needs. Such personnel would function best in an organized setting with proper supervision, training, and assistance.

6. *Rational physician supply.* The number of residencies in specialties in over-supply, such as general surgery, should be sharply reduced. The number of physicians in other specialties and subspecialties where over-supply may be developing (e.g., in the various branches of internal medicine) should be closely monitored. And although we need more physicians to supervise primary care, appeals for heroic increases in the overall supply of physicians should be considered with caution.

7. *Rational hospital utilization.* The danger of overcapacity in community hospitals is more obvious than with respect to physicians. A five-year moratorium on new bed capacity would be salutary, and would provide an opportunity to reassess our medical priorities. Restrictions on bed supply should be accompanied by expansion of home and ambulatory care programs and extended care facilities.

Implementation of these recommendations should have a significant impact on the problems of *cost* and *access.* They should not be expected, however, to produce a dramatic improvement in the overall *health* of the population. Such improvement will more likely come as a result of advances in medical knowledge or of changes in human behavior. By changing institutions and creating new programs we can make medical care more accessible and deliver it more efficiently, but the greatest potential for improving health lies in what we do and don't do for and to ourselves. The choice is ours.

Supplementary Reading

Please see "Stabilizing Health Care's Share of the GDP" in Part 2.

Notes

INTRODUCTION — Health and Economics

1. Gordon McLachan, "From Medical Science to Medical Care," *The Lancet*, no. 7491 (March 25, 1967): 630.

CHAPTER 1 — Problems and Choices

1. Jonathan Spivak, 'Where Do We Go from Here," in Robert D. Eilers and Sue *S.* Moyerman, eds., *National Health Insurance* (Homewood, Ill.: Richard D. Erwin, 1971), p. 272.
2. Raymond Aron, *Progress and Disillusion* (New York: Praeger, 1968), p. 3.
3. R. H. Tawney, *Religion and the Rise of Capitalism* (New York: Harcourt Brace, 1920), p. 270.
4. Henry Sigerist, *Medicine and Human Welfare* (New Haven: Yale University Press, 1941), p. 103.
5. J. Douglas Colman, "National Health Goals and Objectives" (speech delivered to the National Health Forum, Chicago, Illinois, March 20, 1967).

CHAPTER 2 — Who Shall Live?

1. Sigismund Teller, "Birth and Death among Europe's Ruling Families since 1500," in D. V. Glass and D. E. C. Eversley, eds., *Population in History* (London: Edward Arnold, 1965), pp. 87–100.
2. Walsh McDermott, Kurt W. Deuschle, and Clifford R. Barnett, "Health Care Experiment at Many Farms," *Science* 175 (January 7, 1972): 23–31.

3. National Center for Health Statistics, *Comparison of* Neo–Natal *Mortality from Two Cohorts Studies*, Department of Health, Education, and Welfare Publication no. (HSM) 72–1056, Series 20, No. 13 (Rockville, Md., June 1972), p. 8.

4. Herbert G. Birch, "Health and the Education of Socially Disadvantaged Children," *Developmental Medicine and Child Neurology* 10 (1968): 582.

5. National Center for Health Statistics, *Infant Mortality Rates: Socioeconomic Factors*, Department of Health, Education, and Welfare, Series 22, No. 14 (Rockville, Md., March 1972).

6. Dugald Baird, "Infant Mortality and Social Class in Aberdeen, Scotland," *Annual Report of the Association for Crippled Children* (New York: 1971), p. 17.

7. *Infant Death: An Analysis by Maternal Risk* (Washington, DC: Institute of Medicine, 1973).

8. See, for instance, Victor R. Fuchs and Marcia J. Kramer, *Determinants of Expenditures for Physicians' Services in the United States, 1948–1968* (New York: National Bureau of Economic Research, 1972).

9. Walsh McDermott, "Demography, Culture, and Economics and the Evolutionary Stages of Medicine," in E. D. Kilbourne and W. G. Smillie, eds., *Human Ecology and Public Health*, 4th ed. (London: Macmillan, 1969), p. 24.

10. Michael Grossman, "The Correlation Between Health and Schooling," Conference on Research in Income and Wealth, *Household Production and Consumption*, National Bureau of Economic Research, in press.

11. "Unexpected Deaths Increase for Women," *New York Times*, November 20, 1972, p. 34.

12. Grossman, "Correlation Between Health and Schooling."

13. From Sonnet xxix of "Fatal Interview" by Edna St. Vincent Millay. *Collected Poems*, Harper & Row. Copyright © 1931, 1958 by Edna St. Vincent Millay and Norma Millay Ellis. By permission of Norma Millay Ellis.

14. René Dubos, *The Mirage of Health* (New York: Harper, 1959), p. 110.

CHAPTER 3 — The Physician: The Captain of the Team

1. E. F. X. Hughes, E. M. Lewit, R. N. Watkins, and R. Handschin, "Utilization of Surgical Manpower in a Prepaid Group Practice," National Bureau of Economic Research Working Paper 19 (1974).

2. H. G. Mather, N. G. Pearson, *et al.*, "Acute Myocardial Infarction: Home and Hospital Treatment," *British Medical Journal* 3 (1971): 334–338.

3. Eliott Friedson, *Professional Dominance: The Social Structure of Medical Care* (New York: Atherton, 1970), xi.

4. Kenneth Arrow, Uncertainty and the Welfare Economics of Medical Care," *American Economic Review* 53, no. 5 (December 1963).

5. Walsh McDermott, in Edwin D. Kilbourne and Wilson G. Smillie, eds., *Human Ecology and Public Health*, 4th ed. (London: Macmillan, 1969), p. 9.

6. *Ibid.*

7. Sidney Garfield, "The Delivery of Medical Care," *Scientific American* 222, no. 4 (April 1970).

8. William P. Longmire, "Problems in the Training of Surgeons and in the Practice of Surgery," *American Journal of Surgery* 110 (1965): 16.

9. E. F. X. Hughes, V. R. Fuchs, J. E. Jacoby, and E. M. Lewit, "Surgical Work Loads in a Community Practice," *Surgery* 71, no. 3 (March 1972): 315–327.

10. E. F. X. Hughes and E. M. Lewit, National Bureau of Economic Research, paper in progress.

11. This problem was first discussed by Dr. Howard Taylor in connection with the training of obstetricians–gynecologists. See H. C. Taylor, "Objectives and Principles in the Training of the Obstetrician–Gynecologist," *American Journal of Surgery* 110 (1965): 35–42.

12. E. F. X. Hughes, E. M. Lewit, and E. H. Rand, "Operative Work Loads in One Hospital's General Surgical Residency Program," *New England Journal of Medicine* 289 (September 27, 1973): 660–666.

13. Such a plan was introduced by the United Store Workers Union in New York in 1973 in connection with the administration of their health and welfare fund. *New York Times*, June 19, 1973.

14. Department of Health, Education, and Welfare, *Medical Malpractice*, Report of the Secretary's Commission on Medical Practice (Washington, DC: Government Printing Office, January 16, 1973), p. 52.

15. Nathan Hershey and Walter S. Wheeler, "Health Personnel Regulation in the Public Interest: Questions and Answers on Institutional Licensure," California Hospital Association, 1973.

16. See Victor R. Fuchs, Elizabeth Rand, and Bonnie Garrett, "The Distribution of Earnings in Health and Other Industries," *Journal Human Resources* 5, no. 3 (Summer 1970): 382–389. 17. Henry Sigerist, *Medicine and Human Welfare* (New Haven: Yale University Press, 1941), viii.

CHAPTER 4 — The Hospital: The House of Hope

1. Anonymous, "An Interview with J. Douglas Colman," *Hospitals* 39 (April 16, 1965): 45–49.

2. W. John Carr and Paul J. Feldstein, "The Relationship of Cost to Hospital Size," *Inquiry* 4, no. 2 (June 1967): 64.

3. J. Gordon Scannell, *et al.*, "Optimal Resources for Cardiac Surgery," *Circulation* 44 (September 1971), pp. 221–236.

4. John H. Knowles, "The Medical Center and the Community Health Center," in *Social Policy for Health Care* (New York: New York Academy of Medicine, 1969), p. 158.

5. John S. Millis, *A Rational Public Policy for Medical Education and Financing* (New York: National Fund for Medical Education, 1971), p. 104.
6. See Victor R. Fuchs and Marcia J. Kramer, *Determinants of Expenditures for Physicians' Services in the United States, 1948–1968* (New York: National Bureau of Economic Research, 1973).
7. Herbert Klarman, "The Difference the Third Party Makes," *The Journal of Risk and Insurance* 36, no. 5 (December 1969): 553–566.
8. Bernard Friedman, "A Test of Alternative Demand–Shift Response to the Medicare Program" (Paper delivered at the International Economic Association Conference on Economics of Health and Medical Care, Tokyo, April 2–7, 1973).
9. Richard J. Radna, E. F. X. Hughes, and Eugene M. Lewit, "Determinants of Length of Stay in a Group of Neurosurgical Patients" (New York: National Bureau of Economics Research, unpublished).
10. G. R. Ford, "Innovations in Care: Treatment of Hemia and Varicose Veins," in G. McLachlan, ed., *Portfolio for Health* (London: Oxford University Press for Nuffield Provincial Hospitals Trust, 1971).
11. Paul T. Lahti, "Early Post–Operative Discharge of Patients from the Hospital," *Surgery* 63, no. 3 (March 1968): 410–415.
12. Aldolph M. Hutter, Jr., Victor W. Sidel, Kenneth I. Shine, and Roman W. DeSanctis, "Early Hospital Discharge After Myocardial Infarction," *New England Journal of Medicine* 288, no. 22 (May 31, 1973): 1141–1144.
13. Sidney Lee, personal communication.
14. Victor R. Fuchs, "Improving the Delivery of Health Services," *The Journal of Bone and Joint Surgery* 51–, no. 2 (March 1969): 407–412.
15. See Roger G. Noll, "The Consequences of Public Utility Regulation of Hospitals" (Paper delivered at the Conference on Regulation in the Health Industry, Institute of Medicine, Washington, DC, January 7–9, 1974).

CHAPTER 5 — Drugs: The Key to Modern Medicine

1. Allen Norton, *The New Dimensions of Medicine* (London: Hodder and Stoughton, 1969), p. 41.
2. See Reuben Kessel, "Price Discrimination in Medicine," *Journal of Law and Economics* 1 (October 1958): 20–53.
3. J. J. Bums, "Modem Drug Research," in Joseph D. Cooper, ed., *Economics of Drug Innovation* (Washington, DC: American University, 1970), p. 57.
4. Allan T. Demaree, "Ewing Kauffman Sold Himself Rich in Kansas City," *Fortune*, October 1972, pp. 98–103.
5. *The Medical Letter* 15, no. 10 (May 11, 1973): 42–44.
6. *Drug Topics*, March 5, 1973, p. 42.
7. Sam Peltzman, "An Evaluation of Consumer Protection Legislation: The 1962 Drug Amendments," *Journal of Political Economy* 81, no. 5 (September–October 1973): 1049–1091.

8. *Ibid.*
9. Louis Lasagna, "Research, Regulation and Development of New Pharmaceuticals: Past, Present, and Future — Part II," *American Journal of the Medical Sciences* 263, no. 2 (1972): 70.
10. *Ibid.*, p. 72.
11. See W. McVicker, "New Drug Development Study," Industry Information Unit, Food and Drug Administration (Washington, DC: Government Printing Office, 1971).
12. William M. Wardell, "Introduction of New Therapeutic Drugs in the United States and Great Britain: An International Comparison," *Clinical Pharmacology and Therapeutics* 14, no. 5 (September–October 1973): 773–790.
13. William M. Wardell, "British Usage and American Awareness of Some New Therapeutic Drugs," *Clinical Pharmacology and Therapeutics* 14, no. 6 (November–December 1973): 1022–1034.
14. William M. Wardell, "Fluroxene and the Penicillin Lesson," *Anesthesiology* 38, no. 4 (April 1973): 309–312.
15. L. E. Cluff, "Problems with Drugs," Paper presented at the Conference on Continuing Education for Physicians in the Use of Drugs, quoted in Donald C. Brodie, *Drug Utilization and Drug Utilization Review and Control* National Center for Health Services, Research and Development, Department of HEW Publication no. (HSM) 72– 3002 (1971).
16. John M. Firestone, *Trends Prescription Drug Prices* (Washington, DC: Enterprise Institute for Public Policy Research, 1970).

CHAPTER 6 — Paying for Medical Care

1. See Martin S. Feldstein, The Feldstein Plan," in Robert D. Eilers and Sue S. Moyerman, eds., *National Health Insurance* (Homewood, Ill.: Richard D. Erwin, 1971) and "The Welfare Loss of Excess Health Insurance," *Journal of Political Economy* 81, no. 2, part 1 (March–April 1973).
2. Mark V. Pauly, "Discussion of Fein [Rashi] Paper," in Eilers and Moyerman, *National Health Insurance*, p. 108.
3. *Ibid.*, p. 109.
4. Paul M. Elwood, Jr., "Restructuring the Health Delivery System: Will the Health Maintenance Strategy Work?" in *Health Maintenance Organizations: A Reconfiguration of the Health Services System* (Chicago: Center for Health Administration Studies, University of Chicago, May, 1971), p. 3.
5. Ray E. Brown, "Implications of the Health Maintenance Organization Concept," in *Health Maintenance Organizations*, p. 70.
6. August Heckscher, "Medicine and Society," *New England Journal of Medicine* 262, no. 1 (January 7, 1960): 19.

7. Daniel S. Hirschfield, *The Lost Reform* (Cambridge: Harvard University Press, 1970).
8. Jonathan Spivak, 'Where Do We Go from Here," in Eilers and Moyerman, *National Health Insurance*, p. 273.

CONCLUSION — Health and Social Choice

1. John Maurice Clark, "Economic Means — To What Ends?" in *The Teaching of Undergraduate Economics, American Economic Review Supplement* (December 1950): 36.

Part 2
Supplementary Reading

Major Concepts of Health Care Economics

VICTOR R. FUCHS
Stanford University, Stanford CA, USA

This article applies major economic concepts, such as supply, demand, monopoly, monopsony, adverse selection, and moral hazard, to central features of U.S. health care. These illustrations help explain some of the principal problems of health policy — high cost and the uninsured — and why solutions are difficult to obtain.

Health care should be viewed from many perspectives: biological, ethical, political, and economic. The economic perspective is distinct primarily in the concepts that it uses.[1,2] This article applies several major economic concepts to important features of U.S. health care to help noneconomists increase their understanding of current problems of health policy.

The discipline of economics focuses primarily on the operation of a "market-price" economy, so named because the interaction of supply and demand determines the prices (and quantities) of inputs and outputs in markets. Prices serve as signals that influence the behavior of suppliers and demanders. In his seminal book *The Wealth of Nations*, Adam Smith analyzed how such an economy works and argued that this system is the best route to economic success and personal freedom. In his day (1776), most major markets like those for wheat and bread were relatively simple. Today, the markets in some industries are exceedingly complex, and perhaps none more so than in health care.

A primary focus of health care economics is to identify what determines quantity, price, and expenditures (the product of quantity and price). A related goal is to determine whether the quantity, price, or both substantially differ from what

Originally published in *Annals of Internal Medicine*, **162**: 380–383, 2015. Copyright by American College of Physicians.

would prevail if the industry produced the socially most appropriate amount of care at as low a total cost to society as possible. In calculating social costs and benefits, economists include externalities that arise when producers or consumers make choices that do not consider the effects on others, such as the external costs of pollution or the external benefits of vaccination.

For the economist, the optimum circumstance is when the marginal benefit and marginal cost of health care are equal — any greater amount would use resources that could be more beneficial elsewhere. However, this is difficult to assess. There is not one market for health care but many thousands, differentiated by such factors as disease, technology, location, and physician and patient characteristics. In thinking about cost, economists include "opportunity cost," which could be forgone earnings, as an important part of the expense of medical education and training.

SUPPLY

Because supply and demand determine quantity and price, it is useful to identify important special features that affect health care supply and demand in the United States. The prices of many inputs to health care, such as brand-name prescription drugs and specialist fees, are higher in the United States than in peer countries.[3,4] Higher prices for drugs, devices, and equipment (or, more specifically, lower prices in other countries) are primarily the result of central buying in those countries. In economic terms, the quasi-monopoly power that drug manufacturers achieve through patents and marketing is offset in other countries by the monopsony power of governments that typically pay for approximately 75 percent of care.

The U.S. government pays for approximately 50 percent of care but is restrained from negotiating with suppliers for lower prices by legislation and industry lobbying. Physician specialists in the United States sustain higher fees through various organizational devices, including consolidation of practices and professional control of entry, lack of transparency of fees, and the difficulty that patients have in determining the need for and quality of care. Other countries negotiate fees with physicians and control access to specialists to keep expenditures down.

Higher output prices (for procedures, visits, and tests) reflect higher input prices but are also of concern because they vary greatly in what seems to be the same market. They differ among providers in the same market and patients of the same provider.[5] The ability to price-discriminate, that is, to charge different patients different prices for the same service, is prima facie evidence of some monopoly power. Sellers increase profits by setting prices high for buyers who do not have good alternatives and lower for those who do. Mergers and acquisitions have often been a route to greater market control by hospitals. Vertical integration, the merging of hospital and physician groups into a single entity, has also been questioned by antitrust regulators but may cause substantial gains in production efficiency that more than offset any potential increase in monopoly power. Indeed, some of the most efficient care in the country is delivered by organizations that have integrated hospitals, physicians, and insurance.[6]

Determining the most efficient size of an organization to deliver care because of economies of scale is one of the most difficult factors in economic analyses of health care. That a 100-bed hospital is likely to have lower costs than one with 50 beds for similar care is axiomatic because the larger hospital can spread the overhead costs of some central services, such as pharmacy, laboratory, and radiography, over more patients. For care that requires expensive technology and specialized personnel, the economies of scale may justify a much larger hospital. However, greater size often brings greater power to extract a monopoly price from buyers, and in some large hospitals, diseconomies of scale set in as result of difficulties of communication and coordination and escalating costs of administration. That some hospitals can specialize in one kind of care, such as cardiac surgery, to achieve optimal scale and efficiency further complicates the policy problem. Such specialization shifts the burden and cost to general hospitals that must be able to care for all kinds of patients. A hospital's costs increase when it must care for a wide variety of health problems, each with its own optimal scale.

A considerable amount of care in the United States is probably produced at an inefficient scale, particularly if one considers the related problem of failure to use the most efficient combination of inputs. The possibility of substitution among inputs to produce a given output at a lower cost is emphasized by economists but much less so by physicians and others trained in the application of a specialized technology. For the economist, technology influences but does not determine the "best" combination of inputs. The lowest cost for a given quality-adjusted output depends on relative prices of alternative inputs as well as their contribution to production. For example, access to primary care is often discussed in medicine, and some see the only solution as training more primary care physicians. Others recommend more use of nurse practitioners and physician assistants. Still others say that the cost of nurse practitioners has increased so much relative to that of primary care physicians that they are no longer a cost-effective substitute. Dr. Tim Garson has gone one step further in substitutions of inputs by training and employing low-cost "grand-aides" who, supervised by nurse practitioners, provide first-line primary care in the home, especially for elderly patients with multiple chronic problems. In pilot tests in two pediatric Medicaid settings, Garson reported a large decrease in total cost by reducing clinic and emergency department visits.[7]

Output prices are higher in the United States than in other countries partly because of its more complex system of financing and paying for care.[8] Hundreds of insurance companies try to sell their services to millions of employers and persons at substantial administrative expense. Physicians and hospitals incur huge costs in billing many public and private third-party payers and individual patients.

These costs all go into the output prices that determine expenditures for any given quantity of care.

Probably the most important difference in supply between the United States and peer countries is the mix of services offered.[9] In the United States, a higher proportion of physician visits are to specialists or subspecialists. This circumstance would probably result in higher expenditures even if specialist fees were not higher because of greater use of expensive diagnostic and therapeutic interventions.

A related characteristic of supply in the United States that sets it apart from other countries is greater standby capacity. For example, on a per capita basis, persons in the United States receive 2.5 times as many magnetic resonance imaging scans as citizens of the average Organisation for Economic Co-operation and Development country, but the United States has approximately four times as many magnetic resonance imaging machines. Using the ratio of scans to machines in the other countries as a standard, this fact implies a standby capacity in the United States of more than one fourth of these machines. As a result, scans are usually available more quickly and in a more convenient location in the United States than in other countries. The cost of the extra machines, however, adds to expenditures. Lastly, the supply of health care in the United States is more expensive because it includes more privacy, space, and other amenities in hospitals and clinics.

DEMAND

For most persons, the demand for health care is uncertain and utilization is highly concentrated. Although one half of the population has no contact with the health care industry in any given year, approximately 5 percent are said to account for 50 percent of expenditures. Because most persons are risk-averse, a person's uncertainty about demand for health care becomes a demand for health insurance. Another factor also motivates insurance demand: Most persons of moderate or low income prefer to pay for major expenditures (for example, automobiles, refrigerators, and televisions) on a regular monthly basis rather than on a cash basis when they arise.

Health care is often a "big-ticket" item, and health insurance surely is. The annual premium for a family policy currently exceeds $15,000 and often surpasses $20,000. Regular periodic payment, sometimes called "prepayment" in the insurance industry, is particularly useful to many persons when it is automatically deducted from implicit wages and is not available for other spending. The demand for employment-based insurance in the United States is also stimulated by the tax law, which treats the employer's contribution to the premium as tax-free to the employee, although virtually all economists believe that it is simply another form of compensation similar to wages.

A person's demand for health care in the presence of insurance is greater than what it would be without insurance because it lowers the price to the patient.[10]

This effect is labeled "moral hazard." It contributes to higher health care expenditures because it increases the demand for care for any given health status. It may also increase demand by biasing persons against behaviors that protect and enhance health.

Attempts to tinker with the terms of insurance through deductibles and copays are partial offsets to moral hazard, but a 20 percent copay for a $500 procedure just increases the price to $100. Large deductibles with full insurance above a certain level restrain utilization less than advocates claim because patients can accelerate or delay many interventions to take place in the year when the deductible will be met; therefore, the patient faces no cost. Insurance, moreover, cannot be a good explanation for higher expenditures in the United States than in other countries because those countries have more widespread insurance coverage but lower expenditures. Constraints on input prices, a different mix of services, and lower administrative costs in those countries better explain their lower expenditures.

Because patients with pain or other symptoms often do not know the cause of their problem or the interventions necessary to diagnose and treat it, they are susceptible to supplier-induced demand.[11] In a fee-for-service payment system, some health care organizations and individual physicians order diagnostic and therapeutic interventions of doubtful value to increase revenue. This situation can be rationalized by the fact that the insured patient may pay nothing and the intervention may help in defending a malpractice suit. When a particular intervention is widespread in a community, it becomes the standard of care and individual physicians may be loathe not to recommend it regardless of its lack of effectiveness. Changes in methods of reimbursement, such as a shift to capitation payment, could eliminate supplier-induced demand but may induce undertreatment.

One of the biggest potential problems facing voluntary systems of health insurance is the likelihood of adverse selection. Patients typically know more about their potential utilization of care than insurance companies. A premium based on the company's knowledge will be too low to cover the costs of care for high users and will result in a loss. It will be too high for those who expect to be low utilizers and may result in loss of customers. Economics usually concludes that choice is good and more choice is better than less, but this is questionable in the case of health insurance. Some companies will insure only groups of persons to protect against adverse selection of individuals. The mandate for coverage included in the Patient Protection and Affordable Care Act is another effort to solve this problem.

The demand for most goods and services in the United States depends primarily on the willingness and ability of persons or their families to pay, but health care is different because government subsidizes demand by paying for part or all of some patients' care. Sometimes, as with Medicaid, the subsidy is conditional on having a low income. In other cases, as in Medicare, the subsidy is universal, although the government has recently levied a partially offsetting charge on Medicare beneficiaries with incomes above a certain level. Income-tested insurance (for example, Medicaid) helps the poor get care but can induce evasion and avoidance of reported income more than a universal benefit does.

CONCLUSION

This brief survey of major economic concepts applied to important features of health care in the United States sheds light on the principal policy problems: high cost and the uninsured. In the United States, health care expenditures comprise more than 17 percent of the gross domestic product compared with 11 percent in other high-income democracies. The gross domestic product in the United States was approximately $17 trillion in 2014. Thus, the 6-percentage-point difference is $1 trillion. Other countries realize lower costs through a more activist role for government to reduce prices of inputs, simplify the financing and payment of care, and effect a change in output composition to a less-expensive mix. In the United States, despite high expenditures millions of persons remain uninsured even after implementation of the Affordable Care Act. To achieve universal coverage requires subsidies for the poor and the sick and compulsory participation by the entire population.

The Affordable Care Act has introduced substantial changes in health insurance markets but has not made major changes in financing, organization, or delivery of care. Such reform is unlikely for two reasons. First, large-scale change in health care would undoubtedly leave some persons worse off even if most persons would benefit. In the Declaration of Independence, Thomas Jefferson noted the reluctance of people to trade known present problems for uncertain future benefits. Two centuries later, in their Nobel Prize-winning "Prospect Theory: An Analysis of Decision Under Risk," Daniel Kahneman and Amos Tversky argued that most persons give greater weight to a possible loss than to a possible gain of equal magnitude.[12] Moreover, for some persons and groups, the potential losses from health care reform are large and predictable. These potential losers are sufficiently well-financed to be able to use the complex political system in the United States to block major changes. Only a severe political, financial, or medical crisis might make current political calculations and alignments irrelevant and large-scale reform possible.

REFERENCES
1. Culyer, A. J. (2005). *The Dictionary of Health Economics*, Edward Elgar: Northampton, MA.
2. Eatwell, J., Milgate, M. and Newman, P. eds. (1987). *The New Palgrave: A Dictionary of Economics*, 1st edn. Macmillan: London.
3. Cohen, J., Malins, A. and Shahpurwala, Z. (2013). "Compared to US Practice, Evidence-based Reviews in Europe Appear to Lead to Lower Prices for Some Drugs." *Health Affairs (Millwood)* 32: 762–770.
4. Laugesen, M. J. and Glied, S. A. (2011). "Higher Fees Paid to US Physicians Drive Higher Spending for Physician Services Compared to Other Countries." *Health Affairs (Millwood)* 30: 1647–1656.

5. White, C., Reschovsky J. D. and Bond A. M. (2014). "Understanding Differences Between High- and Low-Price Hospitals: Implications for Efforts to Rein in Costs." *Health Affairs (Millwood)* **33**: 324–331.

6. Cutler, D. M., McClellan M. and Newhouse J. P. (2000). "How Does Managed Care Do It?" *The RAND Journal of Economics* **31**: 526–548.

7. Garson, A. Jr, Green, D. M., Rodriguez, L., Beech, R. and Nye, C. (2012). "A New Corps of Trained Grand-Aides has the Potential to Extend Reach of Primary Care Workforce and Save Money." *Health Affairs (Millwood)* **31**: 1016–1021.

8. Cutler, D. M. and Ly, D. P. (2011). "The (Paper) Work of Medicine: Understanding International Medical Costs." *Journal of Economic Perspectives* **25**: 3–25.

9. Fuchs, V. R. (2013). "How and Why US Health Care Differs from that in Other OECD Countries." *The Journal of American Medical Association* **309**: 33–34.

10. Newhouse, J. P. (1982). "A Summary of the Rand Health Insurance Study." *Annals of the New York Academy of Sciences* **387**: 111–114.

11. Fuchs, V. R. (1978). "The Supply of Surgeons and the Demand for Operations." *Journal of Human Resources* **13**(Suppl): 35–56.

12. Kahneman, D. and Tversky, A. (1979). "Prospect Theory: An Analysis of Decision Under Risk." *Econometrica* **47**: 263–292.

Major Trends in the U.S. Health Economy Since 1950

VICTOR R. FUCHS
Stanford University, Stanford CA, USA

Rapid advances in medical science and technology, substantial gains in health outcomes attributable to medical care, and budget-busting increases in health care expenditures fueled by private and public insurance have marked the past six decades of health care in the United States. As the country struggles to emerge from a multiyear financial and economic crisis, policymakers and the public have increasingly homed in on those skyrocketing health care expenditures. What lessons can be drawn from the evolution, since 1950, in the sources of payment and objects of expenditures in the health care arena?

HEALTH EXPENDITURE

The rapid growth of health expenditures is one of the most important economic trends in the United States in the post-World War II era. It has implications for the financial viability of federal and state governments and has resulted in stagnation of wages in most industries. In 1950, health expenditures accounted for only 4.6 percent of the gross domestic product (GDP). In 2009, they accounted for more than 17 percent, a larger share than all manufacturing, or wholesale and retail trade, or finance and insurance, or the combination of agriculture, mining, and construction. According to public finance experts such as Alan Blinder and Alice Rivlin, control of health care expenditures is the greatest fiscal policy challenge facing the United States. From 1950 through 2009, there was an almost continuous increase in annual real per capita health expenditures, with the exception of one 2-year pause in the mid-1990s, when the effect of managed care was at its peak[1] (see Figure 1). The absolute rate of growth has been increasing over time,

Originally published in the *New England Journal of Medicine* **307**(11): 1143–1144, March 15, 2012 ("200th Anniversary Article").

as evidenced by the concave shape of the curve in the graph. The relative rate of increase was greater between 1950 and 1980 than between 1980 and 2009 — 4.6 percent versus 4.1 percent per year — primarily because of the introduction of Medicare and Medicaid in 1965.

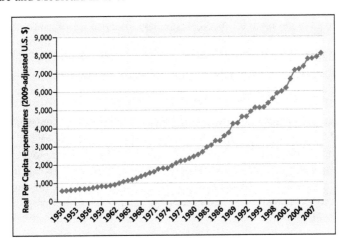

Figure 1
U.S. Per Capita Health Expenditures, 1950–2007.

Unfortunately, the slight slowing in the rate of growth of health expenditures since 1980 was accompanied by even greater slowing in the growth of the GDP (per capita adjusted for inflation), from 2.6 percent per year in 1950–1980 to 1.8 percent per year in 1980–2009. Thus, the gap between the rate of growth of health expenditures and that of GDP increased from 2.0 percent to 2.3 percent per year between the two periods. Most experts believe that such a gap is not sustainable over the long term, because health expenditures would cut too drastically into the availability of other essential goods and services.

The most important explanation for the increase in real per capita health expenditures is the availability of new medical technology[2] and the increased specialization that accompanies it. Between 1974 and 2010 alone, the number of U.S. patents for pharmaceutical and surgical innovations increased by a factor of six. Second in importance is the spread of public and private health insurance, which diminishes the effect of health care prices on demand.[3] There is a positive-feedback loop between new technology and the spread of health insurance: new technology stimulates the demand for insurance, and the spread of insurance stimulates the demand for new technology.[4] Finally, a small portion of the increase, typically 0.1 or 0.2 percentage points per year, is attributable to the aging of the population. It's not possible to estimate how much of the increase in expenditures reflects higher health care prices and how much reflects greater quantities of care, because the content of a day in the hospital or a visit to a physician keeps changing. No doubt some of the increase in expenditures reflects an increase in the quantity of medical care, if quantity is adjusted for improvements in the quality of care.

SOURCES OF PAYMENT

The sources of payment for medical care have changed significantly since 1950 (see Table 1). The most important trends have been a decline in out-of-pocket payment and a rise in third-party payment (both private and public), an increase in government's share of payment and a decrease in the private share, and an increase in the federal government's share as compared with that of state and local governments.

Third-party payment has grown partly because of expensive interventions that expose individuals to large financial risk and partly because employers' contributions to employee health insurance are not considered part of employees' taxable income. Since World War II, there has been a large increase in the number of workers who must pay income tax and an even greater increase in the number who must pay payroll taxes. These increases have made tax-exempt employer-based

Table 1. *Personal Health Care Expenditures in the United States from 1950 through 2009.* *

VARIABLE	YEAR OR PERIOD		
	1950	1980	2009
Per capita expenditures (2009 dollars)	407	2,050	6,807
Source of payment (%)			
Out-of-pocket	56	27	14
Third-party	44	73	86
Private or Public (%)			
Private	73	60	53
Public	27	40	47
Federal	13	26	35
State and local	14	14	12
	1950–1980	1980–2009	1950–2009
Average annual rate of change (% in 2009 dollars)			
Out-of-pocket	3.0	1.9	2.4
Third-party	7.1	4.7	5.9
Private	4.7	3.7	4.2
Public	6.7	4.7	5.7
Federal	7.8	5.0	6.4
State and local	5.2	3.8	4.6

Note: *The percentage of payments by the federal government was calculated on the basis of National Health Care Expenditure data. Data are from the Department of Health and Human Services and the U.S. Census Bureau.

health insurance more attractive. A shift from individual to group insurance has also contributed to the spread of coverage by reducing marketing and administrative costs and, thanks to compulsory participation within firms, limiting the risk of adverse selection for insurance companies.

The growth of government's share, and especially the federal share, can be explained by the public's desire to cover more of the public with insurance and private insurers' difficulty in providing coverage for the elderly and the poor. Federal legislation also substantially extended public coverage for children.

OBJECTS OF EXPENDITURES

Throughout the period since 1950, health expenditures have gone primarily to hospitals, physicians, and drugs. Moreover, the rate of growth of expenditures in each of these categories between 1950 and 2009 has been fairly close to the rate of growth of total health expenditures (see Figure 2). Drug expenditures may appear to have grown more slowly, but that's probably due to a data mismatch: the 1950 figure includes sundries, whereas the 1980 and 2009 figures are for prescription drugs only. Such stability in the share of these categories is remarkable, given the great changes that have occurred in medical technologies, sources of payment, and health policy since 1950. As a rule of thumb, the ratio 3:2:1 does a fairly good job of describing the relative importance (in dollar terms) of hospitals, physicians, and drugs. The "other" expenditures are divided among many categories, the most important of which are public administration and the net cost (premiums minus benefits paid) of private health insurance, nursing homes, and dental services.

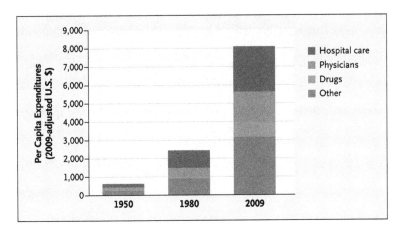

Figure 2

Per Capita Health Care Expenditures in 1950, 1980, and 2009, According to Category.

Source: Data are from the U.S. Census Bureau.

There have been periods in the past 60 years when individual categories accounted for greater or lesser proportions of expenditures. Spending for hospital care and physicians received a boost between 1950 and 1980 from the introduction of Medicare and Medicaid. Spending for drugs accelerated sharply after 1980 following the introduction of a host of new products for treating heart diseases, mental illness, gastrointestinal disorders, and cancer and a large increase in private and public insurance coverage for drugs.

The ability of hospitals to maintain their high share is particularly noteworthy, because between 1950 and 2009 the industry had several large shocks. Psychiatric hospitals virtually emptied out. Admission rates to acute care hospitals ("community" hospitals) dropped precipitously after 1970, as did the average length of stay. As a result, the average daily census, adjusted for population growth, has decreased by almost 50 percent over the past four decades. Hospitals have maintained and increased their revenues in part through more intensive treatment of inpatients. Despite shorter stays, the cost per case (in 2009 dollars) jumped from $6,600 in 1997 to $9,200 in 2009.[5] Hospitals' total incomes were also preserved through expansion of outpatient services, including same-day surgery, magnetic resonance imaging and computed tomography, and outpatient clinics for diagnosing and treating cancer, heart disease, and other illnesses.

COMMUNITY HOSPITALS

Community hospitals (including academic medical centers), the recipients of the largest share of health expenditures, have seen dramatic shifts in demand for and supply of inpatient care since 1950. During the first three decades of this period, the number of inpatient days per 1000 population increased by more than a third, driven by Medicare and Medicaid, the spread of employer-based insurance, and lax utilization controls by public and private payers (see Table 1 in the Supplementary Appendix, available with the full text of this article at NEJM. org). A slight decline in the average length of stay was more than offset by a 50 percent increase in the number of admissions per 1000 population. The industry's 31 percent increase in the number of beds per 1000 population, abetted by consultants' predictions of ever-growing demand, proved to be an expensive mistake. In the late 1960s and early 1970s, there was mounting evidence that many hospital admissions were ill-advised and that lengths of stay for many patients were overly long (see the Supplementary Appendix). Between 1980 and 2009, the number of inpatient days per 1000 population fell by almost half, with declines in admissions and average length of stay contributing almost equally. The decline in length of stay was particularly spectacular in some major categories of patients. For example, stays for uncomplicated myocardial infarction dropped from 3 weeks to 3 days; for uncomplicated vaginal delivery, from 1 week to 1 day; and for herniorrhaphy, from 6 days to same-day surgery. The average decrease among all patients, however, was smaller than those for individual causes of admission, because the average severity of patients' conditions on admission increased. The hospital industry responded to the drop in demand by closing some hospitals (net decrease of 18 percent) and closing off some beds as unavailable, but even so, the average occupancy rate fell by 10 percentage points to the inefficient level of 65.5 percent.

PHYSICIANS

The number of active physicians in the United States increased by a factor of approximately four between 1950 and 2009 (see Table 2 in the Supplementary Appendix). As the population grew, the number of active physicians per 1000 population increased from 1.41 to 2.73, an annual growth rate of 1.1 percent. That figure may overstate the growth of physicians' availability, however, since the number of hours the average physician worked probably decreased appreciably between 1950 and 2009. Major trends in the physician supply that had important implications for the health economy were large increases in the percentages of female physicians, specialist physicians, and hospital-based physicians.

Because women, even professional women, still bear a disproportionate share of domestic responsibilities, female physicians tend to differ from their male peers in preferences regarding annual hours of work, night coverage, self-employment, specialty choice, and other aspects of practice.

The increase in the proportion of physicians who are specialists and subspecialists has resulted in a considerable increase in the number of years the average physician spends in training, although a restructuring of medical education could change that.[6] There has been a large increase in the number of specialists and an even larger increase in the number of specialties and subspecialties, from a few dozen 50 years ago to more than 150 now.

The shift away from office-based practice, along with possible changes in payment systems, may portend a time when most medical care will be delivered by teams of physicians and other health care providers (e.g., nurse practitioners and physician assistants) working in accountable care organizations.

CHANGES IN ORGANIZATION AND DELIVERY

An important recent trend affecting hospitals and physicians is a sharp division between physicians who treat outpatients and others, called hospitalists, who treat only inpatients. The number of hospitalists has grown rapidly, from no more than 1000 15 years ago to 7000 10 years ago to approximately 30,000 in 2011, according to physician-economist David Meltzer of the University of Chicago. Hospitalists are said to improve both the efficiency of care (mostly through reducing lengths of stay) and its quality. Though primary care physicians initially resisted this change in professional responsibilities, many now prefer the new system because they perceive that hospital visits were not an efficient use of their time.

Another trend attracting wide attention is the use of electronic medical records (EMRs) in physicians' offices. Opinions vary regarding the effects of EMRs on the efficiency and quality of care. I believe a well-organized health care system can benefit substantially from EMRs, but the fragmented nonsystem of U.S. medical care is not likely to derive enough benefit to justify the cost.

During this period, another change that affected hospitals and physicians was the development of managed care. Until about 1990, most insured patients could choose freely among providers, physicians' decisions were not subject to frequent questions by insurers, and payment was typically fee for service. The rapid growth of health care expenditures in the late 1980s, combined with sluggish growth of the GDP, fueled a demand for change.[1] In the 1990s, insurers selectively contracted with providers, fees and prices were negotiated in advance, physicians' decisions became subject to insurance-company review, and patients faced financial penalties for obtaining out-of-plan care. The effect on health care expenditures was dramatic: growth rates fell to 2 percent per year by the mid-1990s. At the same time, GDP growth accelerated to about 3 percent per year. Both physicians and patients, however, grew increasingly critical of managed care. Physicians complained about a squeeze on their incomes and interference with their autonomy. Patients resented restrictions on their choice of providers and worried that cuts in spending would necessarily result in a poorer quality of care. The complaint by physicians and patients that health outcomes were adversely affected by managed care, fueled by many anecdotes, has not been supported by systematic evidence.

The term "managed care" still carries negative connotations for many observers, but as long as concern about cost is strong, it's difficult to imagine a widespread call for unmanaged care. Stakeholders will disagree about who should do the managing, about the relative roles of regulation and competition, and what form competition should take. Perhaps the most important future trend, too nascent to quantify, let alone evaluate, is the replacement of the current system of organization and delivery with competition among large accountable care organizations serving defined populations for risk-adjusted per capita annual payments.

PAST AND FUTURE

The six decades since 1950 have been remarkable for the U.S. health economy in many ways, especially the extraordinary increase in health care expenditures. Future historians may, with some irony, refer to this period as a golden age for U.S. medicine because health care's share of the GDP quadrupled from 4.6 percent in 1950 to more than 17 percent in 2009; in most peer countries, the share is 9 to 11 percent. Other noteworthy trends in the health economy have been the spread of private and public health insurance to the point where almost 90 percent of the total bill for care is paid by third parties; the increased role of the federal government in funding health care; the decline in inpatient use of hospitals (fewer admissions and shorter stays) and the expansion of hospital outpatient services; the shift in the physician workforce toward more women, more specialists, and more hospital-based physicians; and the deluge of new medical technologies confronting clinicians with a menu of 6000 drugs and 4000 procedures to choose from.

It is difficult to see how the health sector can continue to expand rapidly at the expense of the rest of the economy, but every past prediction of a sustained slowing of the growth of health expenditures has been proved wrong. Rapid growth may continue as a result of political gridlock regarding the form that curbs on expenditures should take. There is no public consensus about how much care should be provided for the poor and sick or how it should be done. Similarly, there's no public consensus regarding efforts to increase the efficiency of care. A rational approach to the financing, organization, and delivery of care seems politically impossible. However, the observation by de Tocqueville that in the United States "events can move from the impossible to the inevitable without ever stopping at the probable" may prove to be prescient.

Disclosure forms provided by the author are available with the full text of this article at NEJM.org.

REFERENCES

1. Fuchs, V. R. (December 2000). *The Future of Managed Care: Stanford Institute for Economic Policy Research Policy Brief*. Stanford, CA: Stanford University.

2. Pauly, M. V. (2005). "Competition and New Technology." *Health Affairs (Millwood)* **24**: 1523–1535.

3. Newhouse, J. P. (1993). *Free for All? Lessons from the RAND Health Insurance Experiment*. Harvard University Press: Cambridge, MA.

4. Weisbrod, B. A. (1991). "The Health Care Quadrilemma: An Essay on Technological Change, Insurance, Quality of Care, and Cost Containment." *Journal of Economic Literature* **29**: 523–552.

5. Stranges, E., Kowlessar, N. and Elixhauser, A. (November 2011). *Components of Growth in Inpatient Hospital Costs, 1997–2009*, Statistical brief no. 123. Agency for Health Care Research and Quality: Rockville, MD.

6. Fuchs, V. R. (2011). "Alan Gregg Lecture: The Structure of Medical Education — It's Time for a Change." In Presented at the Annual Meeting of the American Association of Medical Colleges, Denver, November 6.

SUPPLEMENTARY APPENDIX
This appendix has been provided by the author to give readers additional information about his work.

Supplement to:
Fuchs, V. R. (2012). "Major Trends in the U.S. Health Economy Since 1950." *The New England Journal of Medicine* **366**: 973–977.

Table 1.   *Short-Stay Acute Care Hospitals (Community Hospitals).*

	1950	1980	2009
Inpatient days (per 1,000 population)	899	1208	633
Admissions (per 1,000 population)	109	159	116
Average length of stay (days)	8.25	7.60	5.43
Beds (per 1,000 population)	3.34	4.37	2.63
Occupancy rate percent)	73.7	75.3	65.5
Outpatient visits (per 1,000 population)	Not available	913	2091

Sources: Statistical Abstract for the United States, 1960, 1990, 2012. Historical Statistics of the United States, From Colonial Times to 1970, Part 1.

1960s–1970s References on Shortened Length of Stay:

Ford, G. R. (1971). "Innovations in Care, Treatment of Hernia and Varicose Veins." In *Portfolio for Health*, ed. G. McLachlan. Oxford University Press for Nuffield Provincial Hospitals Trust: London.

Fuchs, V. R. (1974). *Who Shall Live? Health, Economics, and Social Choice*, Ch. 4. Basic Books: New York.

Hutter, Jr, A. M., Sidel, V. W., Shine, K. I. and DeSanctis, R. W. (1973). "Early HospiDischarge after Myocardial Infarction." *The New England Journal of Medicine* **288**: 1141–1144.

Lahti, P. T. (1968). "Early Post-operative Discharge of Patients from the Hospital." *Surgery* **63**: 410–415.

Table 2.   Active Physicians: Number, characteristics, and regional location.

	1950	1980	2009
Number	219,900[a]	457,500	838,473
Percent			
Males	94%	88%	70%
Females	6%	12%	30%
Primary care	69%	37%	36%
Specialists	31%	63%	64%
Office-based	87%	62%	58%
Hospital-based	13%	38%	42%
Per 1,000 Population			
North	1.69	2.41	3.15
South	1.28	1.75	2.56
Mid West	1.16	1.70	2.18
West	1.46	2.21	2.62

Note: [a]Includes Federal physicians.

Sources: Health — United States, 1982. Statistical Abstract of the United States, 1960, 1965, 1970, 1980, 1990, 2012. Historical Statistics of the United States: From Colonial Times to 1970. President's Commission on the Health Needs of the Nation, Building America's Health, 1953.

The New Demographic Transition: Most Gains in Life Expectancy Now Realized Late in Life*

KAREN EGGLESTON and VICTOR R. FUCHS
Stanford University, Stanford CA, USA

The original "demographic transition" describes a process that began in Europe by the early 1800s with decreases in mortality followed, usually after a lag, by decreases in fertility.[13,28] According to Lee and Recher (2011), p. 1, "this historical process ranks as one of the most important changes affecting human society in the past half millennium." The increase in life expectancy associated with this demographic transition has been accompanied by rising levels of per capita output, which have in turn spurred further improvements in population health through better nutrition and living standards[3,15] and, especially since World War II, through advances in medical care.[12] At the same time, increases in life expectancy have resulted in a higher proportion of each cohort living long enough to participate in the production of goods and services. Reductions in fertility are also closely linked to higher labor force participation rates among women.[11,18,22]

During the original demographic transition, mortality decline prior to fertility decline often led to larger cohorts concentrated in working ages; this transitional change in the age structure of the population provided a boost to income that has been called a "demographic dividend."[6] Swift (2011) documents a significant two-way positive relationship between life expectancy and GDP per capita between 1820 and 2001 for 13 high-income countries.

Now, the United States and many other countries are experiencing a new kind of demographic transition. Instead of additional years of life being realized early

Originally published in *Journal of Economic Perspectives*, **26**(3): 1–22, 2012. Copyright by American Economic Association.

*To access the Appendix, visit http://dx.doi.org/10.1257/jep.26.3.137.

in the lifecycle, they are now being realized late in life. At the beginning of the twentieth century, in the United States and other countries at comparable stages of development, most of the additional years of life were realized in youth and working ages; and less than 20 percent was realized after age 65. Now, more than 75 percent of the gains in life expectancy are realized after 65 — and that share is approaching 100 percent asymptotically. The choice of age 65 to illustrate this new demographic transition is somewhat arbitrary, but if we used 60 or 70 instead, the results would be qualitatively similar.

The new demographic transition is a *longevity* transition: How will individuals and societies respond to mortality decline when almost all of the decline will occur late in life? This issue is broader and more far-reaching than the issue of cohort size in each age group, with its usual focus on the prospective retirement of the unusually large "baby boomer" cohort, and has important socioeconomic implications independent of patterns of fertility.

When the gains in life expectancy occur mainly towards the end of life, they contribute more to the age bracket that is traditionally mostly retired rather than to the age bracket in prime working years. Retirees are highly dependent on transfers from the working population for living expenses, including large consumption of medical care. Thus, gains in life expectancy concentrated at the end of life can unsettle an economy's balance between production and consumption in ways that pose a long-run challenge for public policy. The obvious changes needed (at least "obvious" to many economists) would be to raise productivity, the savings rate, and the age of retirement, but how to accomplish such goals is controversial and uncertain.

This paper covers the years 1900–2007 for the United States and 16 other "developed countries," chosen for the continuity of their mortality data: Australia, Belgium, Canada, Denmark, England and Wales, Finland, France, Iceland, Italy, Netherlands, Northern Ireland, Norway, Scotland, Spain, Sweden, and Switzerland. We focus on demographic statistics including life expectancy at birth and at age 65, the percent of each birth cohort expected to survive to age 65, and the share of the increase in life expectancy at birth realized after age 65. For the U.S. economy, we also calculate expected labor force participation for each birth cohort, which allows us to investigate how changes in mortality affect labor force participation and work-life as a share of life expectancy. Results on the longevity transition and expected labor force participation for the United States and other high-income countries are followed by consideration of economic and social changes in China and other countries that are experiencing an earlier stage of the original demographic transition. The paper concludes with a brief discussion of the long-run implications of the new demographic transition.

THE LONGEVITY TRANSITION

To examine long-term trends in life expectancy at birth, we draw upon the life tables in the Human Mortality Database, which offers high-quality demographic data for selected countries and regions compiled by a respected group of demographers at (http://www.mortality.org). We first extract data on life expectancy at birth; in particular, we calculate "period" life expectancy, which is the projected average age of death for a cohort if it experienced the age-specific death rates prevailing at the year of birth. We also look at rates of survival from birth to age 65 and life expectancy at age 65. We use the five-year period life tables since 1900 (or earliest available year) for each of the 17 countries or regions in the Human Mortality Database that have data extending back at least 70 years. The five-year intervals help to smooth annual fluctuations in demographic trends.

We calculate changes for nine overlapping 20-year intervals: 1907–1927, 1917–1937, and so on up to 1987–2007.* (The years ending in "7" are chosen to represent mid points of each of our five-year intervals.) To calculate the change in years lived past 65, we first multiply survival to 65 by life expectancy at age 65 for each five-year period and then take differences across 20-year intervals. Finally, we calculate the change in years lived past 65 as a percentage of change in life expectancy at birth for each country for each of the nine 20-year intervals.

Figure 1(a) shows that life expectancy at birth has increased almost continuously for well over a century in high-income countries. Much of this rise in life expectancy was due to a particularly large fall in death rates for infants, children, and young adults, resulting in a sharp rise in the percentage of a cohort surviving to age 65, as indicated in Figure 1(b). Survival rates from birth to age 65 more than doubled over the twentieth century from 40.9 percent in 1900–1904 to 83.3 percent in 2005–2009 in the United States. Similarly, survival rates from birth to age 65 in 16 high-income comparators increased from 42.0 to 87.8 percent over the same period.

The other major demographic change that contributes to the longevity transition is an increase in life expectancy at age 65, an increase which has become larger in recent decades as shown in Figure 2(a). The interaction between the increase in life expectancy at age 65 and the increase in the percentage of the cohort that survives to age 65 has resulted in an exceptionally large increase in the share of the gain in life expectancy that is realized after age 65. As can be seen in Figure 2(b), that share was only about 20 percent during each 20-year period at

---

*For our detailed underlying data on the five-year averages for each country, see the online Appendix with this paper at (http://dx.doi.org/10.1257/jep.26.3.137). Online Appendix tables 1–3 show the decreases in the coefficient of variation across the 17 high-income countries for the demographic variables portrayed in Figures 1 and 2. To include data for the United States prior to 1933 (when the Human Mortality Database series begins for the United States), we use life table data from U.S. National Vital Statistics Reports, derived from death registration states for the period 1900 to 1928, and for the whole United States thereafter (all races combined). For a small share of observations at the beginning of the century — Australia, Canada, and Northern Ireland in 1900–1919; Spain in 1900; and the United States in 1905, 1915, and 1925 — we use imputed values from regressions with year and country fixed effects and country-specific linear time trends.

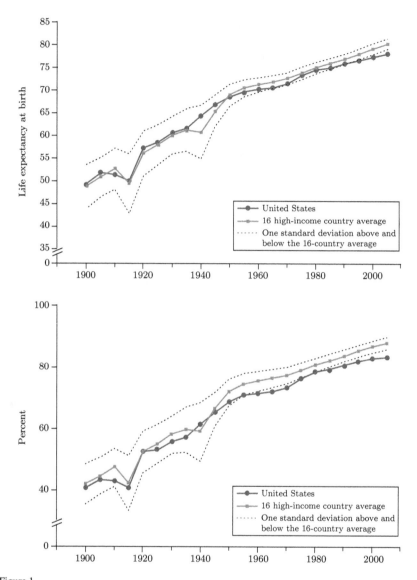

Figure 1

(a) Life Expectancy at Birth and (b) Percent of Birth Cohort Expected to Survive to Age 65, Since 1990 (*in the United States and 16 other high-income countries*).

Source: Authors' calculations using data from the Human Mortality Database and other sources as detailed in the online Appendix.

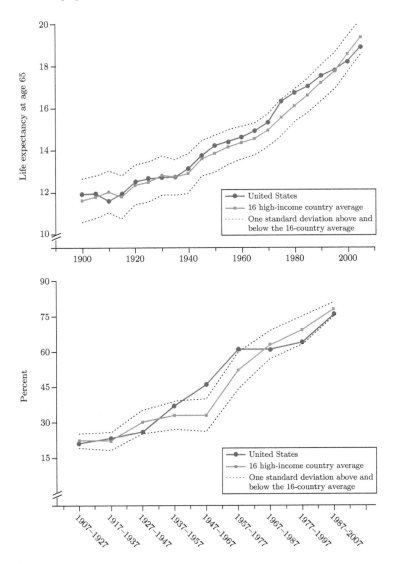

Figure 2

(a) Life Expectancy at Age 65 and (b) Share of Gains in Life Expectancy Realized after Age 65 Since 1990 (*in the United States and 16 other high-income countries*).

Source: Authors' calculations using data from the Human Mortality Database and other sources as detailed in the online Appendix.

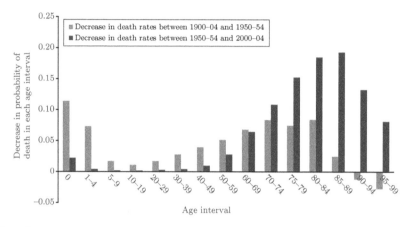

Figure 3

Decrease in Death Rates by Age Group in England and Wales, 1900–1904 to 1950–1954 and 1950–1954 to 2000–2004.

Source: Authors' calculations using data from the Human Mortality Database.

the beginning of the twentieth century, but it was 76 percent in the United States and 78 percent for the 16-country mean by the end of the century, and is approaching 100 percent asymptotically. Our results here are quite similar to, and extend over time, those of Lee and Tuljapurkar (1977) based on the 1995 survival profile of the United States.

We can illustrate the shift in survival improvement toward older ages by comparing the age distribution of mortality decline between the first half and second half of the twentieth century for a region with particularly reliable long-run data: England and Wales. Figure 3 shows that between 1900–1904 and 1950–1954, declines in death rates were largest for infants and children, whereas between 1950–1954 and 2000–2004, declines were most salient for those over age 70. This pattern of age-specific mortality decline across the twentieth century was similar for Sweden, another country where reliable long-run data is available.*

The actual survival of a given birth cohort will differ from the estimates of life expectancy at birth when survival is changing over time. Remember, estimates of life expectancy at birth (what we earlier called "period" life expectancy) are based on the age-specific death rates prevailing at that year of birth. For example, in 1900–1904, life expectancy at birth in England and Wales was 48.6 years.

*For details on Sweden, see the online Appendix. Figure 3 shows a slight increase in death rates for the oldest [90+] age groups between 1900–1904 and 1950–1954, perhaps because of small numbers, less-reliable data, and/or survival of a less-healthy cohort to those ages.

In contrast, the cohort born in 1900–1904 had a cohort life expectancy (actual mean age of death) of 53.8 years, since they experienced part of the increase in survival shown in Figures 1–3. The cohort born only 17 years later experienced a cohort life expectancy of 62.4 years, whereas "period" life expectancy at birth did not reach that level until 1935–1939.[*]

Nevertheless, we find that estimates based on cohort life tables prepared by the Social Security Administration[4] exhibit a similar trend towards survival gains realized late in life: for men, the share of life expectancy increases realized after age 65 was 28 percent between the 1900 and 1920 birth cohorts, rising to a projected 62 percent between the 1980 and 2000 birth cohorts. For women, the share of life expectancy gains realized after age 65 increased from 30 percent (between the 1900 and 1920 birth cohorts) to an estimated 69 percent (between the 1980 and 2000 birth cohorts).

The century-long demographic trends shown in Figures 1 and 2 have been similar in all 17 countries with available data. From a U.S. perspective, the main difference is lagging survival to 65 compared to the other 16 countries (the U.S. line is below the 16-country average in Figure 1(b)); also, the United States experienced a larger rise in female life expectancy at age 65 between the 1940s and 1970s than the other countries. The relative differences among countries have decreased over time, especially for life expectancy at birth and survival to age 65.

THE LONGEVITY TRANSITION AND EXPECTED LABOR FORCE PARTICIPATION

One of the most significant economic effects of the longevity transition is on expected lifetime labor force participation, partly in terms of total years in the workforce and especially in terms of years in the workforce as a fraction of expected years of life. Two factors affecting the connection from life expectancy to years of work are (1) whether the growing numbers of elderly are healthy enough to work and (2) the economic, social, and political pressures for a period of retirement at the end of life.

Greater longevity can have opposing effects on age-specific health status. If improved survival is correlated with reductions in morbidity for the elderly, then illness may be compressed into the end of life, as posited by the "compression of morbidity" hypothesis.[16] On the other side, medical interventions do tend to keep alive those who are in worse health,[47] which suggests the possibility that the longer-lived elderly could be sicker for a longer period. The net effect of rising longevity on age-specific morbidity is an empirical question. According to the National Long-Term Care Survey, the share of elderly Americans with

---

[*]Survival gains have been so dramatic that period and cohort survival significantly differs. For example, age-specific death rates for England and Wales in 1900–1904 would have led to only 43.7 percent of women and 36.4 percent of men surviving to 65. But of the cohort born in 1900–1904, 61.3 percent of women and 49.6 percent of men actually survived to age 65.

severe disabilities decreased from 26.2 to 19.7 percent between 1982 and 1999.[33] Milligan and Wise[35] find a strong within-country correlation between declining mortality and improved self-assessed health for several European countries. Thus, the empirical record suggests that better health in terms of both improved survival and reduced morbidity could tend to raise age-specific rates of labor force participation. Changes in occupational structure which lower the physical demands of work also can increase participation.

Higher incomes tend to increase the demand for leisure, in the form of fewer hours of work per week and, especially recently, as a block at the end of life.[10,37] Furthermore, several factors might give rise to a negative interaction between improved survival and employment, at least for some subgroups. For example, the reduced selection effect of mortality might also increase the proportion of the cohort that is less valued in employment (because of less stamina, ambition, education, and the like), reducing age-specific labor force participation. Alternatively, if firms have pyramid-like organizational structures with many jobs at entry and fewer at higher levels in the hierarchy — such as the military's "up or out" policy regarding age and promotion of officers — then increases in survival will lead to crowding at higher levels of the pyramid and lower rates of participation. Moreover, a sharp rise in employment rates for women, at wages that were often below those paid to men, might have led to some decrease in the demand for men's labor.

On net, which of these forces have predominated over the past century, and which are likely to predominate in the future? Estimates of what we call "expected labor force participation" can help answer this question.

Calculating expected labor force participation

We define "expected labor force participation" (XLFP) as the total years an individual is expected to participate in the labor force, based on period estimates of survival, and labor force participation by gender and age. That is

$$\text{XLFP}_{jt} = \sum_{i=1}^{100} \pi_{ijt} L_{ijt},$$

where L_{ijt} is the labor force participation rate for age i and gender j in year t, weighted by probability of survival to age i (π_{ijt}). It is necessary to examine men and women separately because of the large upsurge in female labor force participation between the 1950s and 2000.[11,20,21] Our calculations rely on labor force participation rates from decennial censuses (1900–1930) and the Current Population Survey (1942–2007). As in the earlier estimates of life expectancy, we can calculate both "period" expected labor force participation, which is based on the age-specific labor force participation rates prevailing at a certain point of time, or the actual realized labor force participation rates for a birth cohort; these estimates will differ when age-specific labor force participation rates are changing over time.

Changes in lifetime expected labor force participation can be decomposed into two factors: changes in survival to given ages and changes in age/sex-specific rates of labor force participation. For example, we calculate the effect of improving survival, holding age-specific labor force participation rates constant at their 2007 values. We also calculate the effect of changing rates of labor force participation, holding survival rates constant.*

Our work is related to the literature on expected lifetime work hours[24] and work-life expectancy,[41] including the work-life estimates for the U.S. population from the 1950s through the early 1980s from the Bureau of Labor Statistics.† As far as we are aware, this paper is the first to produce work-life estimates for the United States covering the period 1900 to 2007, decompose those changes into survival and age/sex-specific labor force participation effects, and to estimate work-life expectancy relative to life expectancy at birth for a broader range of countries in recent decades.

U.S. expected labor force participation since 1900

In the early twentieth century, most of the increase in life expectancy arose from the dramatic decrease in mortality at young ages. This change first increased the years of youth dependency for these cohorts, and then increased expected labor force participation — the expected number of years that an individual will be in the labor force if he or she participates at the average labor force participation rate for each sex and age in a given year.

Figure 4(a) shows that years of expected labor force participation at birth for U.S. males increased by a third — from about 30 to 40 years — between 1900 and 1950. For the most recent half century, however, increases in survival have been offset by decreasing age-specific labor force participation rates for men, causing expected lifetime labor force participation to be relatively constant at about 40 years. Because life expectancy at birth has continued to increase, male expected labor force participation as a fraction of expected years of life has declined, as shown in Figure 4(b). Table 1 shows that in the United States between 1900 and 2000, male labor force participation increased from 30 to 40.5 years, female participation from 6.4 years to 34.4 years, and for the total population from 18.5 to

---

*These are decompositions 1B and 2B, respectively, in Table 7 of the online Appendix. Alternative calculations, using 1900 as the base year (decompositions 1A and 2A), show similar results.

†In other pre-existing work in this area, Hunt and colleagues[26] update worklife estimates for the U.S. based on 1998–1999 labor force participation rates. Reference 36 use a regression framework. In related research, Hazan[24] estimates lifetime working hours for U.S. men born between 1840 and 1970 and for the U.S. population born between 1890 and 1970.

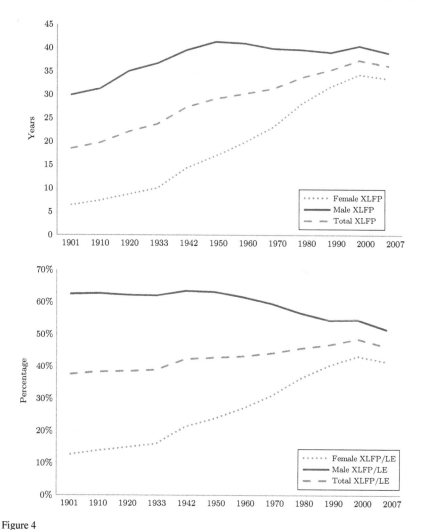

Figure 4

(a) U.S. Expected Labor Force Participation Since 1990 and (b) Expected Labor Force Participation (XLFP) as a Share of Life Expectancy at Birth.

Source: Authors' calculations using data from the Human Mortality Database and other sources as detailed in the online Appendix.

37.4 years. This increase in years of expected labor participation is two-thirds of the total gain in life expectancy at birth of 28.2 years over the twentieth century.

How much of this change is attributable just to longer life expectancies? If we hold age-specific rates of labor force participation constant but allow survival rates to grow at the actually observed pace, the rise in life expectancy alone would have increased expected labor force participation by 13.3 years for males and by 10.8 years for females since 1900 (as shown in Table 1). The effect of mortality decline was concentrated in the first half of the twentieth century. Indeed, for men, if we hold age-specific labor force participation rates constant but allow survival rates to vary in calculating expected labor force participation ("male XLFP holding LFP constant"), the ratio of years of expected labor force participation to life expectancy at birth was relatively constant at 54 percent from early in the twentieth century until about 1970 (not shown in the table). At that point, it began a slow but seemingly inexorable decline, now falling to about 50 percent.

Actual years of expected labor force participation, reflecting both survival effects and changes in age-specific labor force participation rates, have also begun to decline. As shown in both Table 1 and Figure 4(b), the ratio of years of expected labor force participation to life expectancy at birth ($XLFP/LE_0$) has declined for U.S. men from 62.6 percent in 1900 to 51.6 percent in 2007. That same ratio for women increased from 12.7 percent in 1900 to 43.2 percent in 2000, before declining slightly to 41.5 percent by 2007. For the overall U.S. population, years of expected labor force participation divided by life expectancy at birth peaked at 48.6 percent in 2000 and declined slightly to 46.3 percent by 2007.

Table 1. Expected Labor Force Participation in the United States, by Sex, 1900–2007.

	MEN					WOMEN		
YEAR	MALE XLFP	MALE XLFP HOLDING LFP CONSTANT	MALE XLFP ADJUSTED FOR HOURS WORKED	MALE $XLFP/LE_0$	MALE XLFP ADJUSTED FOR HOURS/ LE_0	FEMALE XLFP	FEMALE XLFP HOLDING LFP CONSTANT	FEMALE $XLFP/LE_0$
1900	30.0	25.7	37.28	62.6%	77.9%	6.4	22.7	12.7%
1910	31.3	27.1	39.96	62.8%	80.2%	7.4	24.1	13.9%
1920	35.1	30.4	37.65	62.2%	66.8%	8.7	26.3	14.9%
1933	36.7	32.3	40.40	62.0%	68.2%	10.0	28.3	16.0%
1942	39.5	34.1	42.66	63.5%	68.5%	14.3	30.1	21.3%
1950	41.3	35.6	38.22	63.2%	58.4%	16.9	31.3	23.8%
1960	41.0	36.3	36.79	61.5%	55.2%	19.8	32.0	27.0%
1970	39.9	36.4	34.67	59.5%	51.7%	23.1	32.2	31.0%
1980	39.6	37.4	n.a.	56.6%	n.a.	28.1	32.8	36.3%
1990	39.1	37.9	n.a.	54.4%	n.a.	31.8	33.1	40.3%
2000	40.5	38.7	n.a.	54.5%	n.a.	34.4	33.3	43.2%
2007	39.0	39.0	n.a.	51.6%	n.a.	33.5	33.5	41.5%
Change, 1900 to most recent	9.0	13.3	−2.6	−11.0%	−26.1%	27.1	10.8	28.8%

Table 1. (Continued)

		TOTAL (MEN AND WOMEN)			
YEAR	TOTAL XLFP	TOTAL XLFP HOLDING LFP CONSTANT	TOTAL XLFP ADJUSTED FOR HOURS WORKED	TOTAL XLFP/ LE$_0$	TOTAL XLFP ADJUSTED FOR HOURS/LE$_0$
1900	18.5	24.2	n.a.	37.6%	n.a.
1910	19.8	25.6	n.a.	38.4%	n.a.
1920	22.1	28.4	n.a.	38.5%	n.a.
1933	23.7	30.3	29.0	39.0%	47.5%
1942	27.4	32.2	29.2	42.3%	45.1%
1950	29.1	33.6	29.0	42.8%	42.5%
1960	30.2	34.2	28.8	43.2%	41.2%
1970	31.3	34.4	28.9	44.2%	40.7%
1980	33.8	35.2	n.a.	45.7%	n.a.
1990	35.4	35.6	n.a.	46.8%	n.a.
2000	37.4	36.0	n.a.	48.6%	n.a.
2007	36.3	36.3	n.a.	46.3%	n.a.
Change, 1900 to most recent	**17.7**	**12.0**	**n.a.**	**8.7%**	**n.a.**

Notes: Expected Labor Force Participation (XLFP) is calculated as the total years an individual is expected to participate in the labor force based on period estimates of labor force participation and survival by gender and age. XLFP for a given year represents the expected number of years that an individual would be in the labor force if he or she participates at the average LFP rate for each age in that given year. LE_0 is life expectancy at birth. "XLFP holding LFP constant" uses 2007 age- and sex-specific labor force participation rates, but allows survival to each age to vary as it actually did between 1900 and 2007.

Sources: Author calculations based on survival data from the Human Mortality Database (1933–2007), supplemented by data for death registration states for 1900–1920; and labor force participation rates from decennial censuses (1900–1930) and the Current Population Survey (1942–2007). Adjustments for hours worked draw from Hazan (2009).[24] See the online Appendix for details.

Since 1950, increases in survival and declines in age-specific participation rates of men tended to offset one another. For example, between 1950 and 2007, labor force participation rates of men ages 45–54 declined from 95.8 percent to 88.2 percent, but survival to age 50 increased from 84.1 to 92.2 percent, so the total expected years in the labor force between ages 45 and 55 remained eight years.* For women, increases in years of expected labor force participation mostly

---

*For the detailed data behind these calculations across the range of ages, for both men and women, see online Appendix Table 7, which offers alternative decompositions of changes in both male and female labor force participation. Online Appendix Table 7 also shows that holding age-specific labor force participation rates constant (at either their 1900 or 2007 values) would have led to a larger increase in male expected labor force participation than actually observed.

reflect increases in age-specific rates of labor force participation, especially after 1950. Accordingly, for women, if we hold age-specific labor force participation rates constant but allow survival rates to vary in calculating expected labor force participation ("female XLFP holding LFP constant"), the ratio of years of expected labor force participation to life expectancy at birth has declined slowly but steadily from about 45 percent in the first few decades of the twentieth century to about 40 percent (not shown in the table).

The increase in female labor force participation since the late 1950s could be considered primarily a one-time substitution from unpaid home production to paid work outside the home.[11,21] If so, then the decrease in years of expected labor force participation for women in the United States since 2000 would reflect completion of the one-off change and the beginning of a similar trend as seen for men — that is, a decline of years in the labor force as a share of life expectancy at birth.

Taking into account the decrease in the intensive margin — annual hours worked per full-time worker — tends to reinforce the conclusion that expected work life has declined as a fraction of life expectancy at birth. Hazan[24] estimated lifetime work hours over the past century conditional on survival to age five. We adapt Hazan's data to life expectancy at birth to calculate years of expected labor force participation adjusted for hours worked and show the results in Table 1 (the online Appendix has details of our calculations).

Calculation of a century-long trend in expected years of labor force participation in other high-income countries is not possible because there is no reliable source for internationally comparable labor force participation rates before 1980. Given the similarities in trends of both survival and labor force participation across these countries for the available years, we suspect the trend of declining expected labor force participation as a share of life expectancy at birth that we found for the United States reflects a broad and robust trend that countries experience as they reach high life expectancy levels. Indeed, with the sole exception of the Netherlands, the ratio of years of expected labor force participation to life expectancy at birth has declined since 1980 for males in all other high-income countries in our analyses.* Adjusting for a decline in work hours would reinforce this trend.

DEMOGRAPHIC TRANSITION ACROSS STAGES OF ECONOMIC DEVELOPMENT

The demographic transition traces out a pathway, with many societies arrayed along earlier phases of the transition roughly and imperfectly in accordance with

---

*The online Appendix tables provide calculations of expected labor force participation across 15 countries since 1980; see Appendix Table 8 in the online Appendix available with this paper. Reference 9, p. 17 examines the age at which male mortality was 1.5 percent in 1977 and 2007, finding that at that age almost 90 percent of UK men were employed in 1977, but by 2007, only 30 percent were.

Table 2. The Longevity Transition in Asia and Select Developing Countries.

COUNTRY	CHANGE IN YEARS LIVED PAST 65 AS A PERCENTAGE OF CHANGE IN LIFE EXPECTANCY AT BIRTH, 1990–2010	
	MALES (%)	FEMALES (%)
Japan	72.7	87.0
South Korea	45.4	57.1
China	51.9	40.6
Philippines	26.2	36.0
Indonesia	26.1	35.7
Brazil	34.2	35.0
Vietnam	32.5	34.7
India	23.6	25.8
Bangladesh	20.7	25.4

Source: Authors' calculations based on the life tables for each country prepared by the International Programs Center of the U.S. Bureau of the Census in its International Data Base.

their per capita incomes. Many developing countries are currently experiencing the original demographic transition. For example, Table 2 shows that between 1990 and 2010, the share of years lived past 65 as a percentage of increase in life expectancy at birth was only a little over one-third in Vietnam and Brazil, and less than one-quarter in Bangladesh — comparable to levels a century earlier in today's high-income countries.

Improving health and increasing life expectancy at birth clearly can contribute to better living standards for the world's poor (World Health Organization, 2002). Data on labor force participation for developing countries is not always reliably comparable across countries and over time. Nevertheless, the importance of improved survival for gains in expected labor force participation at early stages of the longevity transition can be illustrated with extant data. For example, in 1980 only 70 percent of Indonesian men survived to age 45; by 2007, 90 percent did. This improved survival added 10 years to expected labor force participation rates for Indonesian males between 1980 and 2007. As a result, expected labor force participation rates for Indonesian males rose to 43.7 years, which was 64.5 percent of life expectancy at birth in 2007.

China and India are especially important cases to consider, given their large populations and relatively rapid economic development. In India, the share of years lived past 65 as a percentage of increase in life expectancy at birth was only one-quarter (as shown in Table 2) in the most recent 20-year period. For China, that share was 52 percent for men and 41 percent for women in the 1990–2010 period.

China's position reflects the rapidity of its demographic transition since the early 1970s and its achievement of relatively high levels of health despite low per capita income by the end of the Mao era.[2,43] Indeed, despite the higher death rates associated with the Great Leap Famine of 1959–1961, China's growth in life expectancy from approximately 35–40 years in 1949 to 65.5 years in 1980 ranks as the most rapid sustained increase in documented global history.[*] These earlier health improvements and growth of the working-age population contributed to China's unprecedented economic growth for the past quarter-century. Wang and Mason (2008) estimate that between 1982 and 2000, about 15 percent of China's rapid growth in output per capita stemmed from the demographic dividend. (Bloom and Williamson (1998) estimate that one-quarter to one-third of the growth rates in the "East Asian miracle" stemmed from the demographic dividend.) Although the pace of mortality decline in China has slowed, it continues: Chinese life expectancy increased between 1990 and 2010 from 69.9 to 76.8 years for women and from 66.9 to 72.5 years for men.

With a rapid demographic transition to relatively low mortality and low fertility, China's population is now aging.[39] Many policy challenges loom as China establishes social and economic institutions commensurate with its transition to a middle-income, market-based economy with a large elderly population.[8,14] One additional challenge for China in reducing the growth-slowing potential of the new demographic transition is China's increasing burden of chronic disease. Fueled by rapid urbanization, increases in high-fat and calorie-rich diets, reductions in physical activity, unabated male smoking and other factors, prevalence of chronic disease in China has quickly caught up with that of high-income countries. For example, the age-standardized prevalence of diabetes among adults in China was 9.7 percent in 2007–2008, more than three times reported prevalence in 1994,[46] comparable to the U.S. rate of 8.3 percent overall in 2010 and 11.3 percent among adults,[9] and higher than the OECD average.[38]

The timing and the rapidity of the longevity transition have varied across countries and regions. For example, in Japan between 1950 and 1970, only 13.1 percent of increase in male life expectancy at birth was realized after age 65; for women, that figure was 17.3 percent. During the 1990 to 2009 period, Japan led the world in the new demographic transition, with the share of gains in life expectancy at birth realized after age 65 reaching 72.7 percent for men and 87 percent for women (again, as shown in Table 2).

---

*Miller *et al.* (2012) assess the relative importance of various explanations proposed for these gains, including better nutrition, widespread public health interventions, improved access to medical care, and increases in educational levels. They find that gains in education and public health campaigns jointly explain 25–32 percent of the crude death rate decline under Mao, and similar proportions of the dramatic reductions in infant and under-five mortality in that period.

The original and the new demographic transitions are inextricably intertwined with the evolution of social and economic institutions.[1] Evidence is mounting that no society at an advanced stage of economic development can presume that further gains in longevity will contribute to growth of per capita income under currently prevailing institutions. For example, Lee and Mason (2011) compare the "average age of consumption" to the "average age of labor income"[*] across a large group of countries for which they and their international collaborators have collected detailed generational accounts, including the value of assets and transfer wealth from social support programs (but not including bequests or value of non-market labor). They find that for developing countries, net transfers flow strongly downward from older to younger ages. However, in a "sea change" analogous to what we call the new demographic transition, "the direction of inter-generational transfers in the population has shifted from downward to upward, at least in a few leading rich nations" including Germany, Austria, and Japan (Lee and Mason, 2011, p. 116). Although the Lee-Mason estimates are cross-sectional, the link to the longevity transition is clear: for the 13 countries that overlap between their dataset and ours, there is a strong negative correlation (−0.89) between the share of gains in life expectancy over the past 20 years that were realized after age 65 and the current number of years by which the average age of income exceeds the average age of consumption. In other words, the more the gains in life expectancy are concentrated in traditional retirement years, the closer the intergenerational transfers are to being upward rather than downward.

For a broader group of 107 countries, Bloom et al. (2010) calculate counterfactual annual growth rates of per capita income between 1960 and 2005, using 2005–2050 projections of demographics. The results vary depending on the level of economic development. They find that in most non-OECD countries, declining youth dependency would more than offset increasing old-age dependency. However, about half of countries would have grown more slowly using 2005–2050 projections of demographics. Among 26 OECD countries analyzed, 25 of them (Turkey is the exception) would have had lower economic growth — averaging 2.1 rather than 2.8 percent per year — under the counterfactual of 2005–2050 demographic change.

POLICY IMPLICATIONS OF THE NEW DEMOGRAPHIC TRANSITION

Historically, adults produced more than they consumed and supported children. With such a pattern in place, the increase in proportion of the population in older years implied by the demographic transition might have been thought to shift out

---

[*]They construct the average ages of consumption and labor income as follows: "The average age of consumption is calculated by multiplying each age by the aggregate consumption at that age, summing these products over all ages, then dividing by the total amount of consumption at all ages. An equivalent calculation gives the average age of labor income" (Lee and Mason, 2011, p. 123).

the social budget constraint as people expanded their number of years worked. However, "a funny thing happened along the way: societies invented retirement ... and the economic consequences of population aging are now viewed with alarm" (Lee and Mason, 2011, p. 115).

Retirement, a relatively new phenomenon in human history, can be viewed as a response to many economic and social changes. Contributing factors include the shift from self-employment on farms or small businesses to wage and salary status; more rapid technological change, resulting in more rapid obsolescence of human capital (alongside compensation packages that often underpay at the beginning and overpay at the end of a career, as discussed in Lazear (1981)); the introduction of a variety of health and welfare programs which assist the elderly but also discourage work; an income-driven increase in the demand for leisure, with the diminishing marginal value of an even shorter work week overtaken by the efficiency gains of a block of leisure at the end of life; and, in times of high unemployment, public concern about job opportunities for younger workers.

Will the new demographic transition inevitably lead to slower economic growth? As people foresee longer lives, they might choose to work longer, save more, and/or invest in human capital in sufficient amounts and innovative enough ways that longer lives continue to contribute to increased prosperity. In this spirit, Bloom *et al.* (2010) assert that "the problem of population ageing is more a function of rigid and outmoded policies and institutions than a problem of demographic change per se" (p. 607).

It is not clear, however, that the United States or other high-income countries even further along in the new demographic transition are reshaping their policies and institutions sufficiently in response to the longevity transition. Although both the United States and France have increased the age of retirement or age to qualify for early retirement, social welfare systems across the high-income countries of the world continue to give strong incentives for earlier, rather than later, retirement.[19] Between 1965 and 2005, the correlation between change in male life expectancy at birth and change in retirement age is actually negative: −0.21 (Bloom *et al.* 2010, p. 591). This trend cannot continue indefinitely: longer and longer retirement lives are not consistent with continued increases in per capita income unless there are significant increases in savings, investment, and productivity. It is ironic that the same phenomenon that led to higher GDP per capita — namely higher life expectancy — could now lead to lower GDP per capita.

Successful navigation of the new demographic transition calls for a combination of policies to give incentives for more savings and investment (including in human capital) earlier in the lifecycle and for additional work later in the lifecycle. Two forces in particular might move the society in that direction: improvement in health, and reductions in the transfers that the elderly can expect to receive from the young.

Public policy should encourage higher labor force participation for the elderly, both by reducing the disadvantages that employers face when employing older workers and by providing enhanced incentives to individuals to continue to work. "People cannot expect to finance 20–25 year retirements with 35-year careers," Shoven noted.[23] "It just won't work. Not in Greece [or] the United States. ... Eventually, we are going to have to increase retirement ages." However, increasing labor force participation for the 65-plus age group alone probably won't make a big difference: even a doubling of those rates from their 2007 levels of 12.6 for women and 20.5 for men would not bring the U.S. ratio of expected labor force participation to life expectancy at birth back to its 2000 level. Increased labor force participation by men in the 50–64 age bracket is also needed.

Public policy might also seek to improve productivity, with an emphasis on education and building human capital early in the lifecycle, and on investment to reduce morbidity and improve the ability to work later in life. Whether compression of morbidity later in life will continue depends on whether improvements in medical technology and in the socioeconomic determinants of health are offset by adverse trends such as increasing obesity. A potentially promising focus here would be to consider investments in public health and medical technologies that reduce morbidity and improve quality of life, as well as more focus on medical innovations that reduce costs of care. (One example of a policy consistent with both objectives would be expansion of palliative care as a substitute for what can otherwise be extremely expensive end-of-life care in a hospital — especially in countries where the concept of hospice services is relatively new, such as China.)

Finally, increased savings, investment, and capital formation could help in fueling endogenous growth.[32,40] U.S. personal savings rates have been low for many decades. Increasing the savings rate of individuals before they retire would ameliorate the potential adverse impact of longevity on economic growth. Countries will need to make fiscally realistic structural changes to entitlement programs — such as Medicare and Social Security in the United States — to support acceptable living standards and improvements in health.

High-income societies are now facing a new demographic transition: the longevity transition. They must decide how to respond to mortality decline when almost all of the decline will occur late in life. Additional increases in life expectancy will result in further declines in expected labor force participation as a percentage of life expectancy at birth unless there is a significant rise in labor force participation rates across both middle and older ages. Of course, increased life expectancy has great value independent of its relationship to per capita income.[37] The original demographic transition gave society a "demographic gift" of higher per capita incomes[7] without much need for a policy response, but the new demographic transition requires politically difficult policies if societies wish to preserve a positive relationship running from increased longevity to greater prosperity.

REFERENCES

1. Aoki, M. (2011). "The Five-Phases of Economic Development and Institutional Evolution in China and Japan." Presidential Lecture at the 16th World Congress of the International Economic Association.
2. Banister, J. (1987). *China's Changing Population.* Stanford University Press: Stanford, CA.
3. Barker, D. J. (1990). "The Fetal and Infant Origins of Adult Disease." *British Medical Journal* **301**(6761): 1111.
4. Bell, F. C. and Michael, L. M. (2005). *Life Tables for the United States Social Security Asia 1900–2100.* Actuarial Study No. 120, Social Security Administration Office of the Chief Actuary, SSA Pub. No. 11–11536. http://www.socialsecurity.gov/OACT/NOTES/s2000s.html.
5. Bloom, D. E., Canning, D. and Fink, G. (2010). "Implications of Population Ageing for Economic Growth." *Oxford Review of Economic Policy* **26**(4): 583–612.
6. Bloom, D. E., Canning, D. and Sevilla, J. (2003). *The Demographic Dividend: A New Perspective on the Economic Consequences of Population Change.* Monograph Reports, MR-1274. RAND Corporation: Santa Monica, CA. http://www.rand.org/pubs/monograph_reports/MR1274.
7. Bloom, D. E. and Williamson, J. G. (1998). "Demographic Transitions and Economic Miracles in Emerging Asia." *World Bank Economic Review* **12**(3): 419–455.
8. Chen, Q., Eggleston, K. and Li, L. (2011). "Demographic Change, Intergenerational Transfers, and the Challenges to Social Protection Systems in China." *Demographic Transition and Inclusive Growth in Asia.* Edward Elgar: Cheltenham, UK.
9. Centers for Disease Control and Prevention (CDC) (2011). "National Diabetes Fact Sheet, 2011." CDC: Atlanta, GA. https://www.cdc.gov/diabetes/library/factsheets.html.
10. Costa, D. L. (1998). *The Evolution of Retirement: An American Economic History, 1880–1990.* University of Chicago Press: Chicago, USA.
11. Costa, D. L. (2000). "From Mill Town to Board Room: The Rise of Women's Paid Labor." *Journal of Economic Perspectives* **14**(4): 101–122.
12. Cutler, D., Deaton, A. and Lleras-Muney, A. (2006). "The Determinants of Mortality." *Journal of Economic Perspectives* **20**(3): 97–120.
13. Davis, K. (1945). "The World Demographic Transition." *Annals of the American Academy of Political and Social Science* **237**(1): 1–11.
14. Eggleston, K. N. and Tuljapurkar, S. eds. (2010). *Aging Asia: Economic and Social Implications of Rapid Demographic Change in China, Japan, and South Korea.* Shorenstein APARC; distributed by Brookings Institution Press: Washington, DC.
15. Fogel, R. W. (1994). "Economic Growth, Population Theory and Physiology The Bearing of Long-term Processes on the Making of Economic Policy." *American Economic Review* **84**(3): 369–395.
16. Fries, J. F. (1980). "Aging, Natural Death, and the Compression of Morbidity." *New England Journal of Medicine* **303**(3): 130–135.
17. Fuchs, V. R. (1999). "Provide, Provide: The Economics of Aging." In *Medicare Reform: Issues and Answers*, eds. A. J. Retten-maier and T. R. Saving. University of Chicago Press: Chicago, USA, pp. 15–36.
18. Galor, O. and Weil, D. N. (1996). "The Gender Gap, Fertility, and Growth." *American Economic Review* **86**(3): 374–387.
19. Gruber, J. and Wise, D. A. (1998). *Social Security Programs and Retirement around the World.* University of Chicago Press: USA.
20. Goldin, C. (1986). "The Female Labor Force and American Economic Growth: 1890 to 1980." In *Long-Term Factors in American Economic Growth,* Conference on Income and Wealth, Volume 51, eds. Stanley Engerman and Robert Gallman. University of Chicago Press: USA, pp. 557–604.
21. Goldin, C. (1990). *Understanding the Gender Gap: An Economic History of American Women.* Oxford University Press: New York.

22. Guinnane, T. W. (2011). "The Historical Fertility Transition: A Guide for Economists." *Journal of Economic Literature* **49**(3): 589–614.

23. Haven, C. (2011). "Stanford Economist: How Do We 'Get off This Path of Deficits as Far as the Eye Can See?'" *Stanford Report,* August 2. http://news.stanford.edu/news/2011/august/shoven-debt-qanda-080211.html.

24. Hazan, M. (2009). "Longevity and Lifetime Labor Supply: Evidence and Implications." *Econometrica* **77**(6): 1829–1863.

25. Human Mortality Database. University of California, Berkeley and Max Planck Institute for Demographic Research. www.mortality.org.

26. Hunt, T., Pickersgill, J. and Rutemiller. H. (2001). "Recent Trends in Median Years to Retirement and Worklife Expectancy for the Civilian U.S. Population (Prepared Using 1998/99 BLS Labor Force Participation Rates)." *Journal of Forensic Economics* **14**(3): 203–227.

27. Lazear, E. P. (1981). "Agency, Earnings Profiles, Productivity, and Hours Restrictions." *American Economic Review* **71**(4): 606–620.

28. Lee, R. D. (2003). "The Demographic Transition: Three Centuries of Fundamental Change." *Journal of Economic Perspectives* **17**(4): 167–190.

29. Lee, R. D. and Reher, D. S. (2011). "Introduction: The Landscape of Demographic Transition and Its Aftermath." *Population and Development Review* **37**(Issue Supplement s1): 1–7.

30. Lee, R. D. and Mason, A. (2011). "Generational Economics in a Changing World." *Population and Development Review* **37**(Issue Supplement s1): 115–142.

31. Lee, R. D. and Tuljapurkar, S. (1997). "Death and Taxes: Longer Life, Consumption, and Social Security." *Demography* **34**(1): 67–81.

32. Lucas, R. E. (1988). "On the Mechanics of Economic Development." *Journal of Monetary Economics* **22**(1): 3–42.

33. Manton, K. G. and Gu, X. (2001). "Changes in the Prevalence of Chronic Disability in the United States Black and Nonblack Population above Age 65 from 1982 to 1999." *Proceedings of the National Academy of Science of the United States of America* **98**(11): 6354–6359.

34. Miller, N. G., Eggleston, K. N. and Zhang, Q. (2012). "Understanding China's Mortality Decline under Mao: A Provincial Analysis, 1950–1980." Unpublished paper.

35. Milligan, K. and Wise, D. A. (2011). "Social Security and Retirement around the World: Historical Trends in Mortality and Health, Employment, and Disability Insurance Participation and Reforms — Introduction and Summary." NBER Working Paper 16719.

36. Millimet, D. L., Nieswiadomy, M., Hang, R. and Slottje, D. (2003). "Estimating Worklife Expectancy: An Econometric Approach." *Journal of Econometrics* **113**(1): 83–113.

37. Murphy, K. M. and Topel, R. H. (2006). "The Value of Health and Longevity." *Journal of Political Economy* **114**(4): 871–904.

38. OECD (2011). *Health at a Glance 2011: OECD Indicators.* Organization for Economic Cooperation and Development: Paris, France. http://www.oecd.org/dataoecd/6/28/49105858.pdf.

39. Peng, X. (2011). "China's Demographic History and Future Challenges." *Science* **333**(6042): 581–587.

40. Romer, P. M. (1990). "Endogenous Technological Change." *Journal of Political Economy,* **98**(5), Part 2: *The Problem of Development: A Conference of the Institute for the Study of Free Enterprise Systems,* pp. S71–S102.

41. Smith, S. J. (1982). "New Worklife Estimates Reflect Changing Profile of Labor Force." *Monthly Labor Review* **105**(3): 15–20.

42. Swift, R. (2011). "The Relationship between Health and GDP in OECD Countries in the Very Long Run." *Health Economics* **20**(3): 306–322.

43. Wang, F. (2011). "The Future of a Demographic Overachiever: Long-Term Implications of the Demographic Transition in China." *Population and Development Review* **37**(Supplement): 173–190.

44. Wang, F. and Mason, A. (2008). "The Demographic Factor in China's Transition." In *China's Great Economic Transformation,* eds. L. Brandt and T. G. Rawski. Cambridge University Press: Cambridge, MA, pp. 136–166.
45. World Health Organization (2002). *Macroeconomics and Health: Investing in Health for Economic Development: Report of the Commission on Macroeconomics and Health:* World Health Organization WHO: Geneva.
46. Yang, W., Lu, J., Weng, J., Jia, W., Ji, L., Xiao, J., Shan, Z., Liu, J., Tian, H., Ji, Q., Zhu, D., Ge, J., Lin, L., Chen, L., Guo, X., Zhao, Z., Li, Q., Zhou, Z., Shan, G. and He, J. (2010). "Prevalence of Diabetes among Men and Women in China." *New England Journal of Medicine* **362**(12): 1090–1101.
47. Zeckhauser, R. J., Sato, R. and Rizzo, J. (1985). "Hidden Heterogeneity in Risk: Evidence from Japanese Mortality." In *Health Intervention and Population Heterogeneity: Evidence from Japan and the United States.* National Institute for Research Advancement: Tokyo, Japan, pp. 23–131.

Social Determinants of Health: Caveats and Nuances

VICTOR R. FUCHS
Stanford University, Stanford CA, USA

Belief in the importance of the social determinants of health is gaining wide acceptance; this useful development will undoubtedly contribute to better public policy and clinical practice.[1] Although the general concept is not contested, several caveats and nuances should be considered.

First, statements such as "social determinants explain half the variation in health" are neither correct nor incorrect; they are incomplete. Assessments of the relative importance of different determinants depend critically on the health variation to be explained. For instance, if the goal was to explain the sharp increase in life expectancy at birth in the United States during World War II, 0.5 percent per annum from 1940 to 1945, health determinants could be divided roughly into 3 categories: social (eg, income, education, neighborhood), biological (genes), and medical care (quantity and quality, including state of science and technology). Significant biological changes over such a short period as World War II did not contribute to increase in life expectancy. Absent any major scientific or technological change and the diversion of approximately half of all practicing physicians to military service during the war, medical care would be an unlikely explanation. That leaves social determinants such as unusual increases in income, decreases in unemployment, and positive shifts in the national psyche inspired by war as the most likely explanations.

Another example of variation is the rapid decline in cardiovascular and cerebrovascular mortality between 1970 and 1980. Again, the period is too short for biological change to have played a role. Some social changes such as a decrease in smoking among men likely contributed. However, smoking among women did

Originally published in *JAMA*, **317**(1): 25–26, January 2017. Copyright by American Medical Association.

not decrease, but vascular mortality among women declined at the same rate as among men. The most likely explanation is medical care, especially more aggressive and effective control of blood pressure. Before the Veterans Administration multisite studies of 1967 and 1970, a systolic blood pressure of 100 mm Hg plus the patient's age was considered normal and did not require treatment.[2,3] As noted in the fourth Joint National Committee,[4] by extending the Veterans Administration practices to other patient populations, gains in hypertension control contributed to a 50 percent decline in coronary artery disease mortality.[4]

A third example is low infant mortality among Mexican Americans, with a rate slightly less than the rate among non-Hispanic whites.[*] That this could be explained by more or better-quality medical care is unlikely. The percentage of people without health insurance is above average for Mexican Americans, who often live in medically underserved areas. Similarly, the social conditions for Mexican Americans, as reflected in income and education, are worse than for non-Hispanic whites. That leaves a biological explanation as the likely explanation.

When discussing the relative importance of social determinants and medical care for health outcomes, a critical distinction must be made between cross-sectional variation in health at a point in time and changes in health outcomes over time. In studies across states, cities, and other geographical regions, differences in the quantity of medical care are easily controlled for, and the frontier of medical science and technology is, for all practical purposes, similar everywhere. For such cross-sectional variation, the social determinants, such as income, education, and neighborhood and health behaviors such as cigarette smoking, usually provide more explanatory power than differences in medical care. By contrast, variation in health outcomes over time in the United States at present is usually explained more by advances in medical science and technology. In recent decades, some social determinants such as a decline in cigarette smoking have contributed to better health outcomes, but some, such as an increase in the prevalence of obesity and the fragmentation of families, have had the reverse effect. Social determinants, as a group, probably explain little of the increase in life expectancy.

In understanding the relative importance of social determinants or medical care in increasing life expectancy over time, it is vital to specify where and when. In the United States in the early decades of the 20th century, before the discovery and diffusion of antibiotics, life expectancy increased rapidly, primarily because of improved sanitation, cleaner drinking water, and improving living standards. Medical care did not have a significant role in the rate of increase of life expectancy from 1900 to 1930 of 3.1 years per decade. By contrast, the increase in life expectancy in the most recent 30 years of 1.5 years per decade was attributable

*US Department of Health and Human Services (HHS) Office of Minority Health. Infant mortality and Hispanic Americans. HHS website. http://minorityhealth.hhs.gov/omh/browse.aspx?lvl4&lvlid68. Accessed October 24, 2016.

less to social determinants than to better control of high blood pressure and cho-
lesterol levels, substantial advances in perinatal interventions, and superior diagnostic and therapeutic interventions for patients with trauma.

A large number of social variables-income, education, housing, nutrition, occupation, and others-are correlated with life expectancy, and most are highly correlated with each other. This multicollinearity increases the difficulty of allocating
scarce resources to derive the most health benefit. The answer may depend on the
particular health problem being addressed. For example, if the goal is to close the
gap in life expectancy between Black and white populations, the most effective
interventions may be different from those for closing the gap between rural and
urban populations.

Chetty *et al.*[5] have documented a substantial correlation between income and
life expectancy derived from millions of individual observations, but they decline
to conclude that this proves a causal mechanism from income to life expectancy.
An alternative inference is a causal mechanism from health (life expectancy) to
income. Moreover, it is possible that the causal connection runs one way at certain
socioeconomic levels and reverses at another.

Years of schooling completed has a strong negative correlation with the probability of smoking, which is highly correlated with life expectancy. But a study
of the probability of smoking at age 17 years (when all individuals in the study
had approximately the same amount of schooling) revealed an equally high negative correlation between the probability of smoking and years of schooling the
individual would have completed by age 24 years. This is evidence against the
hypothesis that additional years of schooling is the cause of the differential in the
probability of smoking.

Some health outcomes may vary as the result of interactions between 2 or more
determinants. Research on such interactions between the genes of individuals and
interventions of medical care are proceeding at a rapid pace. But the possibility
of interaction with social determinants should also be considered. For example,
for a given diagnosis, the appropriate choice between treatment with surgery or
medication might depend on the social condition of the patient. Similarly, the best
policy choice of public health interventions might depend on the social determinants of the target population.

The increasing recognition by the health care community of the importance of
social determinants of health along with biological and medical care is welcomed.
The embrace of these insights, however, should be accompanied by an awareness
that the relative importance of different determinants depends on the variation in
health to be explained. Application of these insights to public health and clinical
policies will improve as more is learned about the causal mechanisms between
determinants and health, of interactions between determinants, and the size as
well as the direction of effects on health.

REFERENCES

1. Adler, N. E., Glymour, M. M. and Fielding, J. (2016). "Addressing Social Determinants of Health and Health Inequalities." *The Journal of American Medical Association* **316**(16): 1641–1642.

2. Veterans Administration Cooperative Study Group on Anti-hypertensive Agents. (1967). "Effects of Treatment on Morbidity in Hypertension: Results in Patients with Diastolic Blood Pressures Averaging 115 Through 129 mm Hg." *The Journal of American Medical Association* **202**(11): 1028–1034.

3. Veterans Administration Cooperative Study Group on Anti-hypertensive Agents. (1970). "Effects of Treatment on Morbidity in Hypertension II: Results in Patients with Diastolic Blood Pressure Averaging 90 Through 114 mm Hg." *The Journal of American Medical Association* **213**(7): 1143–1152.

4. 1988 Joint National Committee (1988). "The 1988 Report of the Joint National Committee on Detection, Evaluation, and Treatment of High Blood Pressure." *Archives of Internal Medicine* **148**(5): 1023–1038.

5. Chetty, R., Stepner, M., Abraham, S. *et al.* (2016). "The Association Between Income and Life Expectancy in the United States, 2001–2014." *The Journal of American Medical Association* **315**(16): 1750–1766.

6. Farrell, P. and Fuchs, V. R. (1982). "Schooling and Health: The Cigarette Connection." *Journal of Health Economics* **1**(3): 217–230.

The Structure of Medical Education — It's Time for a Change

VICTOR R. FUCHS
Stanford University, Stanford CA, USA

Last spring, in his elegant commencement address to the Harvard Medical School, Dr. Atul Gawande appealed for a dramatic change in the organization and delivery of medical care. His reason, "medicine's complexity has exceeded our individual capabilities as doctors." He accepts the necessity of specialization, but he criticizes a system of care that emphasizes the independence of each specialist. Dr. Gawande is not alone in thinking that scientific, technologic, and economic changes require reorganization of care. Larry Casalino and Steve Shortell have proposed Accountable Care Organizations (ACOs); Fisher, Skinner, Wennberg and colleagues at the Dartmouth Medical School have focused on reforming Medicare, and many others have also called for major changes.

I expressed similar concerns in 1974 in my book *Who Shall Live?* but at that time I rejected the claim that the problems of medical care had reached crisis proportion. In 2011, however, I agree with those who say the need for comprehensive reform must be marked URGENT. The high and rapidly rising cost of health care threaten the financial credibility of the federal and state governments. The former finances much of its share of health care by borrowing from abroad; the states fund health care by cutting support of education, maintenance of infrastructure, and other essential functions. These are stopgap measures; neither borrowing from abroad nor cutting essential functions are long-run solutions. The private sector is equally distressed. Surging health insurance premiums have captured

Originally the Alan Gregg Lecture was presented at the Annual Meeting of the Association of American Medical Colleges, November 6, 2011; and printed in *More Health Care Reform*, Stanford, CA: SIEPR, 2012.

most of the productivity gains of the past 30 years, leaving most workers with stagnant wages. Not only is there a pressing need for changes in organization and delivery, but Ezekiel Emanuel and I, in our proposal for universal vouchers funded by a dedicated value-added tax, argue that such changes must be accompanied by comprehensive reform of the financing of medical care (Brookings paper).

But that's not what I want to talk to you about today. My subject is the urgent need to change the structure of medical education. It seems to me that such change is necessary, and perhaps inevitable, given the revolution in medicine over the past half century, and given the changes in organization and delivery of care that lie on the horizon.

THE NEED FOR CHANGE

Consider the deluge of new medical technologies in recent decades. According to Dr. Gawande, in deciding on interventions for their patients, clinicians now must choose from 6,000 drugs and 4,000 procedures. To be sure, many of the 6,000 are not new chemical entities but rather combination drugs, alternative dosage forms, and other variations. Still, the burden on the clinician to make an appropriate choice is great, especially if, as stated in the Physician Charter, "physicians are required to provide health care that is based on the wise and cost-effective management of limited clinical resources." Economists have been touting cost-effectiveness for years, but it is a harbinger of change to see organizations representing more than half of all active physicians sign a charter committing them to practice cost-effective medicine.

Along with the new technologies, there has been a proliferation of specialties and subspecialties. Fifty years ago, there were 18 specialty boards and very few subspecialties. Now there are 36 specialty boards and 116 subspecialty certifications, for a total of 152. Does such proliferation provide much or any benefit to patients? The United Kingdom has only 97, while Canada and France have fewer than half as many. Proliferation of specialties and subspecialties almost certainly adds to the cost of medical education and the cost of care, while its effect on quality of care has not been systematically investigated. The former chair of medicine at a major academic medical center thinks it has an adverse effect on patient care, but other experts disagree. We just don't know the answer. If empirical studies conclude that so many subspecialties are desirable, the training structure that produces them should and could be made more efficient. Medicine is one of the few fields that requires specialists to have more training than generalists. This may have been rational at one time, but may not be today.

Finally, and closely related to the new technologies and increased specialization, there is the soaring cost of medical care. In 1960 U.S. health expenditures, in 2009 dollars, were $864 per person. In 2009, they were $8085. Along with the cost of medical care, the cost of medical education has increased exponentially.

In the face of such revolutionary changes, how has the structure of medical education adapted? It seems that the answer is hardly at all. Fifty years ago, the basic structure was 4 years of college, 4 years of medical school, and 3 years of post-graduate training. Only after 11 years of post-high school graduation was the physician deemed ready to practice medicine. The same is true today, although a much larger percentage than formerly go beyond 11 years to obtain additional specialized training. And in one medical school I know of, fewer than 40 percent graduate in 4 years.

THE GOALS OF CHANGE

A reasonable goal for structural reform might be to reduce that basic period from eleven to nine years. This can be done by cutting time off the front end or the back end of the process or both. About the front end, I note that there are now 33 medical schools that combine college and medical training in 6 years. Could there be more such schools? What is known about the quality of care delivered by physicians from these programs compared with the graduates of conventional medical schools? Very little. Most other developed countries combine college and medical school in one program that is typically less than 8 years long. Are their physicians inferior to American physicians?

It might be argued that foreign medical schools can admit students directly from high school because the educational achievement of those high school graduates is greater than that of American high school graduates. This is probably true on average, but there are certainly some American high school graduates with educational achievement equal to those who graduate from foreign high schools. Why couldn't American medical schools consider for admission applicants who, through appropriate examinations and interviews, appear to be as well qualified as the college graduates the schools are now admitting, regardless of how many post-high school years the student has completed? I understand that thoughtful leaders in medicine are studying various possibilities for accelerating admission to medical school for qualified candidates. That's great. But I hope they realize that the health care system is entering the "ICU," prompt, decisive action is needed.

In order to reduce time at the back end, schools might consider accelerating choice of specialization. Dr. Gawande notes that there was a time when "doctors could hold all the key information patients needed in their heads and manage everything required themselves." He says that in such a world it made sense for physicians to prize "autonomy, independence, and self-sufficiency." But that time is gone forever. What remains is a structure of medical education based on those outmoded assumptions. For Dr. Gawande, who is as handy with a metaphor as with a scalpel, the bottom line is "we train, hire, and pay doctors to be cowboys. But it's pit crews people need."

A PROPOSED NEW STRUCTURE

If Dr. Gawande is correct, what does this imply for the structure of medical education? Isn't it time to give up the conventional wisdom that pouring more and more knowledge into each physician about more and more subjects will produce a better system of medical care? Far from rejecting specialization, embrace it sooner. For the purpose of stimulating discussion, I propose the following structure for medical education:

- Two years of medical education taken by all students. This common curriculum would consist of 50 percent basic science with an emphasis on competencies that would be useful to every physician. Subsequent exposure to basic science would depend on its relevance to the student's prospective career.
- One-third of the time would be devoted to an introduction to clinical care of individual patients, making as full use as possible of modern technologies that have been successful in training programs in industry, the armed forces, and other settings.
- One-sixth of the time would be used to cover key aspects of the health of populations and the organization and delivery of care, with emphasis on a team approach to enhance health. It is important for all physicians, regardless of prospective careers, to understand how each element fits into a health care system.

Upon completion of the 2 years, each student would select a track which launches him or her into the world of specialization. Here is an example of what the tracks might look like:

- Leaders of primary care teams, possibly sub-divided into adult care, pediatric care, and geriatric care.
- Clinical specialists in medicine, hospital based and ambulatory.
- Clinical specialists in surgery and other procedural specialties.
- Possibly another track for those headed for specialties such as radiology and pathology that treat medical and surgical patients.
- A track for students whose major interest is research, possibly similar to current MD-PhD programs but with explicit recognition that the trainees are not preparing to be clinicians.

The content of the training program would differ depending on the track. For example, students training to be leaders of primary care teams would be exposed to more statistics, epidemiology, preventive medicine, and management skills than those in the other tracks. They would learn how to deploy nurse practitioners, physician assistants, and other non-physicians most effectively.

Is it feasible for students to make specialty decisions sooner than they do in the present structure? Before you answer with a resounding "no," let me tell you a "tale of two schools."

A TALE OF TWO SCHOOLS

Just a stone's throw from the Stanford School of Medicine (if you have a good arm) is the Stanford School of Engineering. The latter school accepts students after they have completed 2 years as undifferentiated Stanford undergraduates. Prospective students of engineering are encouraged to take a wide variety of courses during their first 2 years at Stanford, but are also advised to make sure they are getting a good start toward engineering through courses in mathematics and science. At the beginning of their junior year the engineering students declare which of 17 fields they plan to specialize in. The fields range (alphabetically) from Aeronautics and Astronautics to Product Design and include such well-known specialties as Chemical, Civil, Electrical, and Mechanical Engineering.

Notice that the choice of specialization is made 2 years after high school graduation. I may have said that too rapidly. Let me repeat it. Two years after high school, engineering students at Stanford commit themselves to one of 17 specialties. At MIT students must choose their specialty at the end of their freshman year. The heavens do not fall. The SAT scores of the engineering students suggest that they are intellectually about equal to the Stanford medical students. The School of Engineering helps students learn about the various specialties by offering 20 seminars on different subjects with enrollment preference given to freshmen. Examples of seminar subjects are: "Bioengineering Materials to Heal the Body," "Digital Dilemmas," "Water, Public Health and Engineering," and "What Is Nanotechnology?" An additional 12 seminars are offered on other subjects with enrollment preference given to sophomores. Examples of their titles are: "Electric Automobiles and Aircraft," "Environmental Regulation and Policy," "Medical Device Innovation," and "The Flaw of Averages." These seminars provide an opportunity to work closely with faculty. In addition there are many one-unit seminars that provide exposure to key issues and current research in various fields. At the end of 4 years at Stanford, approximately 80 percent of the engineering students graduate with a bachelor's degree and enter the workforce to practice their specialty. Students who go on for a fifth year typically do so in order to earn a master's degree.

There are of course, many differences between engineering and medicine. Biologic systems are probably more complex than the systems engineers work with, and causal relations are less firmly established. An alleged difference is that physician decisions affect life and death, but the same could be said for many engineers. The men and women responsible for our bridges and tunnels, the design of our airplanes and cars, the safety of our water supply, and many similar functions are surely making decisions that affect life and death. One of the biggest differences is that engineers specialize from the start of their training; they are not expected to know about all aspects of engineering. They typically work in team settings. They are, to use Dr. Gawande's words, "pit crews" not "cowboys." Collectively, they get the job done. Perhaps the biggest difference is that when a

medical student chooses a specialty, he or she is usually choosing a life-time occupation. For an engineering student, life-time occupation is not as closely linked to
choice of specialty training. One reason for persistence by physicians in a certified
specialty is that diminished competition affords the specialist the opportunity to
earn a "monopoly rent."

TRAINING SUBSPECIALTIES

As an example of how specialty training in medicine does not have to take
as many years as tradition demands, consider Dr. Robert Chase's experience in
training plastic surgeons at Stanford. When he began his program, plastic surgery
required completion of residency in general surgery followed by another residency program in plastic surgery. The combination took a minimum of 7 years
and more often eight or nine. Drawing on his experience as chief resident in general surgery at Yale, a two-year fellowship in plastic surgery at the University
of Pittsburgh, and active duty in the Valley Forge Army hospital, Dr. Chase was
pretty sure he could train plastic surgeons in no more than 6 years and often in
four or five. To this end he developed an integrated program that started residents
headed for plastic surgery side by side with residents headed for general surgery.

The idea was rejected by the American Board of Plastic Surgery, but he pursued
it anyway. Fortunately, the first residents to complete the program did so well at
both the written and oral examinations that the Board gave tentative approval to
the program. Today there are 27 truly integrated programs similar to Stanford's,
and another 62 that combine general and plastic surgery; only 27 of the traditional
programs remain. It would be surprising if similar shortening could not be accomplished in other fields of medicine and surgery. What is required is an exceptional
clinician-teacher who is willing to confront the established powers and prospective specialists who are willing to commit sooner to their specialty.

ARGUMENTS AGAINST AND OBSTACLES TO RESTRUCTURING

Until now, medical education has proceeded under the premise that "Keeping
one's options open" is a free good. It is not; and the costs to the individual and
society increase every year. Those who set the rules and requirements must consider the possibility that what their generation had to endure may not be the best
path for the future. Many of the existing rules and requirements seem to be based
only on "tradition." The same academic physicians who would not prescribe a
drug without determining efficacy and safety, have no hesitancy in prescribing the
structure of medical education without any studies that examine the appropriateness of that structure relative to alternatives.

Changing the structure of medical education will not be easy, even for those
who are enthusiastic about the goal. Opponents will be numerous, and the arguments varied. Many of the most popular ones are not persuasive. Consider the
cliché, "If it ain't broke, don't fix it." The existing structure may not be "broke,"

but it provides the intellectual foundation for a medical care system that is causing the rest of the country to go broke. Some will say that my suggestions are "controversial." I agree. For more than fifty years I have observed and participated in attempts to reform college curricula, and I can tell you that reforms that are not controversial are inconsequential. Some will want to take credit for the gain in life expectancy of 8.4 years over the past half century. But other developed countries with different systems of medical education and medical care have achieved even greater gains and are at a higher level, while their per capita spending on medical care is 35 to 50 percent less.

Two possible objections to changes discussed in this lecture are that they threaten the deeply held (albeit antithetical) visions of the physician as scientist and the physician as humanist. The threats are real, but the visions are increasingly unreal. American medical education is at a cross-road: Shall it continue to strive to produce scientists-humanists or recognize that what society needs most at this time are competent professionals, capable of providing leadership and supervision for the more than 15 million individuals now employed in the delivery of health services. The challenge to the leaders of medical education is to figure out what kind of admission policy and what structure and content of medical education, undergraduate and post-graduate, will produce such professionals at a reasonable cost. It could be correctly argued that the cost of medical education is a relatively small part of the total cost of medical care, so why change medical education? The reason is that a restructured admission policy, earlier specialization, and shorter period of training can contribute to producing a different physician, one better suited for a team approach to remedying the cost, access, and quality problems now evident in American health care.

The obstacles to change will be partly external to the medical education establishment and partly internal. Consider, for example, the dense network of laws and regulations that now govern the practice of medicine. Some are federal, most are state, and often differ from one state to another. Those that are worth preserving should be federalized. These laws and regulations have been passed with the present structure of medical education in mind. Change in that structure will require changes in the existing legal framework. Many of the laws were enacted with the stated purpose of "patient protection," but as is true in so many industries, they often wind up giving providers protection from competition.

Consider also how malpractice attorneys will leap on health outcomes that fall short of ideal and try to tie these lapses to changes in medical education. We badly need a better system of dispute resolution to replace malpractice suits. Consider also, how large insurance companies and hospitals will resist change, not necessarily because the change would harm them in the long run, but because change is usually disruptive and costly in the short run.

Perhaps the biggest obstacle to change will be within the medical education establishment which includes not only the medical schools but also post-graduate training programs and the bodies that control certification for 152 specialities and subspecialties. Are all these necessary? Restructuring will undoubtedly require some faculty to change what they do and some faculty may be redundant. Many specialty and subspecialty boards will need to change their criteria, as in the case of plastic surgeons. In some areas it may be difficult at first to find medical educators well-equipped to meet the needs of students in the new structure. For instance, where will medical schools find instructors to train the students who have opted for the track of leaders of primary care teams?

Finally, there is the chicken or the egg problem. There are medical leaders who see the need for significant changes in the financing, organization, and delivery of care. But they feel stymied by the absence of physicians with the preparation and attitudes necessary to be most effective in the new systems of care. There are leaders in medical education who see the need for significant changes in structure and content, but wonder where the graduates of the new programs will find appropriate employment.

All these obstacles suggest that restructuring may be impossible. But I draw some hope from an observation made by Alexis de Toqueville who said, "The United States moves from the impossible to the inevitable without ever stopping at the probable."

This is the end of my jeremiad. If I have offended any in the audience, I apologize. That was not my intent. I have, for many decades, studied the American health care system, focusing on the high cost, the inequalities in access, and the lapses in quality of care. I concluded that these problems will not yield to piecemeal reforms. What is needed is comprehensive change in the financing, organization, and delivery of care.

But I have not paid much attention to medical education. Dr. Gawande's Harvard commencement address made me realize that reform of the health care system must be accompanied by a restructuring of medical education. Hence this lecture. Perhaps my suggestions for restructuring are off the mark. Some in this audience may have better ideas as to how it should proceed. If so, all to the good. If I have convinced you of the urgency of the task and stimulated you to address the problem, my effort will not have been in vain. I greatly appreciate the opportunity you have afforded me, and I thank you for your patience.

I await your questions with interest and a reasonable amount of apprehension.

The Doctor's Dilemma — What Is "Appropriate" Care?

VICTOR R. FUCHS

Stanford University, Stanford CA, USA

Most physicians want to deliver "appropriate" care. Most want to practice "ethically." But the transformation of a small-scale professional service into a technologically complex sector that consumes more than 17 percent of the nation's gross domestic product makes it increasingly difficult to know what is "appropriate" and what is "ethical." When escalating health care expenditures threaten the solvency of the federal government and the viability of the U.S. economy, physicians are forced to reexamine the choices they make in caring for patients.

In an effort to address this issue, physicians' organizations representing more than half of all U.S. physicians have endorsed a "Physician Charter" that commits doctors to "medical professionalism in the new millennium." The charter states three fundamental principles, the first of which is the "primacy of patient welfare." It also sets out 10 "commitments," one of which states that "while meeting the needs of individual patients, physicians are required to provide health care that is based on the wise and cost-effective management of limited clinical resources." How can a commitment to cost-effective care be reconciled with a fundamental principle of primacy of patient welfare?

The dilemma arises for two main reasons. First, recent decades have witnessed a flood of new, expensive medical technologies (drugs, imaging devices, surgical procedures) that are of varying degrees of value to patients. A few are true breakthroughs, with strong favorable effects on mortality and morbidity. Others make a meager contribution, at best, to health outcomes. Moreover, technologies that may provide high value for carefully selected patients are often used indiscriminately

Originally published in *New England Journal of Medicine* **365**(7): 585–587, August 2011.
Copyright by Massachusetts Medical Society.

for a much larger cohort of patients. Second, health insurance, private or public, has become so widespread that 90 percent of the country's health care bill is paid by third parties, not by the patient receiving the service.

What is a conscientious physician to do? Some new cancer drugs cost thousands of dollars per month for a single patient. The bills for many surgical procedures run to five or even six figures. Noninvasive imaging devices can offer information to assist in diagnosis, at a cumulative cost in the billions of dollars. U.S. patients, on average, get almost three times as many magnetic resonance imaging scans as Canadian patients; there is no evidence that this large differential can be explained by national differences in the medical condition of patients or that it results in significant national differences in health outcomes. So what level of utilization deserves to be called "appropriate"?

If insurance were not widespread, many physicians would be reluctant to order an expensive intervention unless it offered a good chance of substantial benefit — that is, unless it was cost-effective. Indeed, without U.S.-style cost-insensitive insurance, many expensive diagnostic and therapeutic innovations would not be developed and brought to market.[1] The insured patient, on the other hand, will usually want any and all care that might possibly be of net benefit, regardless of cost. The physician may recognize that the intervention under consideration is not cost-effective but may recommend it anyway, for a variety of reasons: to keep the goodwill of the patient, to protect against a malpractice suit, or in the belief that the "primacy of patient welfare" makes the denial of such care "inappropriate" and "unethical."

The doctor's dilemma is the nation's problem. Some policy experts think that if patients had "more skin in the game" — that is, had less insurance — the problem would be solved. It would not. Even the most ardent advocates of deductibles and copayments acknowledge the need for an annual cap on patients' payments, beyond which insurance takes over completely. There is no consensus on the right level for the cap, but it is generally recognized that the average U.S. household, with large debts and minimal financial assets, could not handle much more than $5,000. But the extreme skew in annual health care expenditures, with 5 percent of individuals accounting for 50 percent of spending in any given year, means that many health care decisions, and especially those involving big-ticket interventions, will be made by and for patients whose costs have exceeded the cap.

Another popular "solution" is to eliminate care that does more harm than good — that is, "unnecessary" care. Such elimination would be desirable, but the potential savings from this source are smaller than is usually claimed. It is true that after the fact, many interventions turn out to be useless or even harmful for some patients. But the heterogeneity of patient populations and uncertainty about the response of individual patients to an intervention means that it is often difficult or impossible to determine in advance which ones will prove to help particular patients and which will turn out to have been unnecessary.

There is no escaping the fact that many interventions are valuable for some patients even if, for the population as a whole, their cost is greater than their benefit. Under what circumstances are they likely to be ordered, and when are they likely to be withheld? The context within which the physician practices, his or her assumption about the behavior of other physicians, and the economic and health consequences of ordering all the care that might do some good versus practicing cost-effective medicine will affect the physician's choice. If the physician is paid on a fee-for-service basis and the patient has open-ended insurance, the scales are tipped in favor of doing as much as possible and against limiting interventions to those that are cost-effective. In that setting, who would benefit from the resources that are saved by practicing cost-effective medicine is not obvious to the physician.

In contrast, if the physician is practicing in a setting that has accepted responsibility for the health of a defined population and the organization receives an annual fee per enrollee, the chances of the physician's practicing cost-effective medicine are substantially increased, even though all patients are insured. The physician's colleagues are practicing the same way, and the resources saved can be used for the benefit of the defined population, which includes the physician's patient. In Canada, which has universal insurance, per capita spending on health care is only 55 percent of the U.S. level because there is a limited overall budget, and all physicians in the system recognize the need for prudence in making decisions about care.

In short, when physicians are collectively caring for a defined population within a fixed annual budget, it is easier for the individual physician to resolve the dilemma in favor of cost-effective medicine. That becomes "appropriate" care. And it is an ethical choice, as defined by philosopher Immanuel Kant, because if all physicians act the same way, all patients benefit.[2]

REFERENCES

1. Weisbrod, B. (1991). "The Health Care Quadrilemma: An Essay on Technological Change, Insurance, Quality of Care, and Cost Containment." *Journal of Economic Literature* **29**: 523–552.
2. Kant, I. (1949). *Critique of Practical Reason and Other Writings in Moral Philosophy*, trans. L. W. Beck. University of Chicago Press: Chicago.

How to Save $1 Trillion Out of Health Care

VICTOR R. FUCHS
Stanford University, Stanford CA, USA

Americans spend more than 17 percent of GDP on health care; other high income industrial democracies spend only about 11 percent. The 6 percent difference in our $17 trillion economy amounts to $1 trillion.

The excess in the United States is primarily attributable to a more expensive mix of procedures and services, higher prices paid to drug companies and physicians, and inefficiencies in the financing of health care. There are undoubtedly cultural differences between the United States and other countries, but it is also true that Swedes differ from Italians, Germans from French, and the English from all of the above.

What these countries have in common that distinguishes their health care systems from the American is universal insurance for basic care, a larger share of government in financing health care (typically about 75 percent of the total versus 50 percent in the United States), and more aggressive control of expenditures.

What could Americans do with that trillion dollars each year and what would we have to give up if our health care system became more like those of our peers?

In the United States, the private sector pays about one-half of the health care bill; federal, state and local governments pay the other half. Assuming the same split in savings from a more prudent system, the private sector could keep half of the trillion dollars for consumption and investment, while the other half could be used for public investment. For example, $500 billion could:

- Increase expenditures on highways, bridges, tunnels, and other infrastructure by 50 percent. Annual cost: $100 billion.
- Increase annual salaries of K-12 teachers by an average of $25,000. Annual cost: $100 billion.

Originally published in the *New York Times*, March 14, 2014.

- Fund a two-year apprenticeship program for one million men and women ages 17–24. Annual cost $80 billion.
- Provide a first-class pre-school experience for all four-year olds. Annual cost: $80 billion.
- Provide additional teachers for arts, music, math and physical education in K12 and expand counseling in high schools. Annual cost: $70 billion.
- Fund R&D for renewable sources of energy. Annual cost: $40 billion.
- Fund R&D for waste disposal (including nuclear) and reduction of pollution. Annual cost: $20 billion.
- Fund after school sports programs for young people 8–18. Annual cost: $10 billion.

To free a trillion dollars from health care, what would we have to give up? The answers come from statistics compiled by the Organization for Economic Cooperation and Development, which includes 34 countries, mostly advanced industrial democracies, that I used to compare United States health care with the *average* OECD country.

- Fewer visits to specialists and a higher proportion of physician visits to primary care providers.
- A sharp reduction in the number of high-tech procedures such as MRI and CT scans.
- A reduction in aggressive medical interventions for the very sick elderly.
- Longer waits for access to specialized care and high tech interventions except for emergencies.
- Less privacy, space, and amenities for in-hospital patients. The number of beds per capita would actually increase as would the number of physicians.

Would these changes have a significant effect on health outcomes? Probably not. Differences in life expectancy between and within developed countries depend more on genes, psycho-social and physical environments, socio-economic factors, and personal behaviors (smoking, diet, exercise) than on differences in health care expenditures.

Tradeoffs like these might attract many Americans, probably a majority. But there are individuals and groups that would clearly be made worse off by such changes. Profits would fall for manufacturers of drugs, devices, and equipment. High-income physician specialists would face substantial reductions in fees and fewer opportunities for specialty training and practice. Hospital revenue would fall. Many smaller insurance companies would be redundant. The loss of prompt access to specialists and high-tech diagnostic and therapeutic interventions and the reduction in privacy and amenities in hospitals might be particularly missed by higher income patients.

Although a majority of Americans might favor the tradeoffs, the political prospects for reallocating the trillion dollars are not good. The United States political system, with its separate houses of Congress and an independent executive branch, augmented by expensive primary battles and long election campaigns, provides many "choke points" for special interests to block or reshape legislation. Escalation in their lobbying and financial contributions also has a significant influence on health policy. In the absence of a severe political or financial crisis, the United States probably will continue to ignore the potential trillion-dollar tradeoff.

DRUGS: THE KEY TO MODERN MEDICINE

Preface to "Innovation and Shortage: The Yin and Yang of the Health Sector"

In Professor Victor R. Fuchs' 1996 Presidential Address to the American Economic Association, he recommends the United States establish "a large private center for technology assessment financed by a small industry-wide levy on all health spending," arguing that such a technology assessment center would be necessary to "help to contain costs without the imposition of controls or caps that might stifle innovation and progress."[*] The following article focuses on this dilemma of trading off innovation and cost control, while upholding what Professor Fuchs also argued in the conclusion of *Who Shall Live*: "elementary justice seems to require greater equality in the distribution of medical care."[†]

The pleasure and honor of a lifetime has been collaborating with some of the luminaries of the health economics field, such as Professor Fuchs. I have also had the honor of coauthoring with several of my Harvard mentors (e.g., Joseph Newhouse, Richard Zeckhauser), including the world-renowned Hungarian scholar of socialism compared to capitalism, János Kornai. The following excerpt (from an article published as part of a special issue honoring Kornai) offers a mildly provocative hypothesis about innovation and shortage in health care. "Shortage" simply means that demand exceeds supply at the given price. Prices are not used to determine who receives numerous goods and services, as Roth (2015) and others have discussed; few societies have a "free market" for human organs, for example.[‡] A chronic shortage of kidneys or hearts is not addressed through higher prices. Chronic shortage is one of the inherent features of many non-market

---

[*] "Economics, Values, and Health Care Reform," *American Economic Review* **86**(1): 1–24; quotes from *Who Shall Live* Second Expanded Edition, pp. 212 and 217.

[†] *Who Shall Live* Second Expanded Edition, p. 149.

[‡] Roth, Alvin E. (2015). *Who Gets What — and Why: The New Economics of Matchmaking and Market Design*. Houghton Mifflin Harcourt.

systems, including centrally planned economies, or "classical socialism" (Kornai 1992).* Accordingly, I argue in this article that a comparative economic systems perspective can enrich our understanding of health policy.

Karen Eggleston,
July 2022

---

* Kornai, János (1992). *The Socialist System: The Political Economy of Communism.* Princeton University Press.

Innovation and Shortage: The Yin and Yang of the Health Sector

KAREN EGGLESTON
Stanford University and NBER,
Stanford CA, USA

INTRODUCTION

In the 21st century, economies will increasingly face the challenge of innovating to address "shortage within surplus" in a vital sector of the economy — that of health and medical care. This sector is growing as a share of the economy in virtually all countries, and the dilemmas of balancing innovation for longevity with solidarity in distribution will be exacerbated by genomic and proteomic "precision and personalized medicine" (PPM) breakthroughs.

In Chinese philosophy, Yin and Yang often represent contradictory yet inseparable opposites — two forces that not merely co-exist, but are synergistic and mutually dependent. This concept is an apt analogy for the relationship between innovation and shortage in the health sector.[*]

INNOVATION AND SHORTAGE

Innovation and its determinants form the centerpiece of *Dynamism, Rivalry, and the Surplus Economy* by János Kornai (2013), a significant contribution to our understanding of the two major economic systems of the past two centuries, socialism and capitalism. Shortage characterizes centrally-planned economies. Lack of innovation is both the cause and result of this phenomenon of socialist systems: "The shortage economy, one of the strongest system-specific properties of socialism, paralyzes the forceful engine of innovation, the incentive to fight for the favors of the customer.... The producer/seller is not compelled to attract the buyer by offering him a new and better product [or service], since the latter is

Originally published in *Acta Oeconomica*, **68**(s1), 99–114, 2018.

[*]This similarity of health sectors with shortage economies, unless carefully understood for its linkage to innovation, might exacerbate the tendency of some — especially in the US — to decry "socialized medicine." To the contrary, organized financing with embedded income solidarity and risk solidarity is integral to enabling our society to sustain a stream of health technology innovations that improve our well-being and longevity.

happy to get anything..., even an obsolete and poor-quality product [or service]" (Ref. 1, p. 15).

However, shortage can appear in specific sub-sectors of capitalist economies as well; indeed, "phenomena of shortage appear universally in the allocation and utilization of free or almost-free public services" (Ref. 1, p. 125). Health economists will recognize the concept of moral hazard, how health systems cope with imbalance of supply and demand, and the "dynamic moral hazard" from insurance coverage that spurs innovations.

To the extent that shortage is inextricably linked to the social impulse to provide equitable access and solidarity in life chances, this phenomenon has its bright side. As emphasized in the literature on the origins of inequality, opportunities for education and self-fulfillment depend on a child's luck of birth in a poor or rich country[2]; and those born into socialist regimes during the 20th century usually benefited from the enhanced access to basic health technologies that such systems promoted:

> The socialist state's paternalist pricing policy and financing of the welfare sectors exert equalizing effects, which ultimately involve a redistribution of incomes. Practically everybody is entitled in a shortage economy to free public education and free health care, including poorer strata that would not be able to pay their cost in a "pure" market economy (Ref. 1, p. 112).

Indeed, East Germany's life expectancy at the lowest quintile exceeded that of West Germany for much of its existence; and China's largest increases in life expectancy occurred under the Mao-era socialist system.[3]

Numerous measures that substantially enhanced length and quality of life in resource-constrained economies included population health campaigns and addressing basic social determinants of health for the vulnerable segments of the population. In some instances, technological breakthroughs also took place under socialism. For example, artemisinin combination therapy is the standard combination therapy for one of worst global killers, malaria, and derives from a traditional Chinese medicine treatment. Artemisinin (青蒿素, Qinghaosu) treatment for malaria was discovered (1972) and manufactured (1979) as part of a military project initiated under Mao Zedong's government (project 523) in China; in 2009 it was approved by the US Food and Drug Administration; and earned discoverer Youyou Tu first the prestigious Lasker-DeBakey Clinical Medical Research Award, and then the Nobel Prize in Physiology or Medicine in 2015.[4]

However, as will be discussed below, this example may be the exception that proves the rule that Kornai argued, the lack of a socio-economic context for breakthrough technological innovations and their marketization in economies characterized by general shortage. It is also important to acknowledge the limits to our knowledge about how best to promote institutional innovation. Necessity may be the mother of invention, but invention does not always spring to life whenever it appears to be a necessity, as the premature mortality throughout the low-income world attests. Moreover, the institutional innovation that socialist countries were adept at promoting — low-cost population health measures relying on individuals to comply with centralized orders — do not appear to be the most salient for breakthroughs in health in the 21st century. Societies are still struggling with how best to promote individual healthy behavior, and post-socialist economies have not been any more effective than traditionally capitalist ones — indeed, in many cases considerably less successful — in convincing individuals to quit smoking, stop excessive drinking, eat healthily, and avoid sedentary lifestyles that lead to premature mortality. Moreover, while substantial health gains could follow from such simple measures as consistent use of seatbelts and bicycle/motorcycle helmets, the technological innovations extending life in the 21st century may derive more from personalized therapies for cancer and cardiovascular disease.

INNOVATION AND SHORTAGE: YIN AND YANG IN THE HEALTH SECTOR

The health sector is everywhere shaped by the dynamic interaction of innovation and shortage, while dealing with numerous market failures in health care financing and delivery.[5] The seemingly inexorable increases in healthcare spending are driven by innovations: "The rate of health care spending growth cannot exceed income growth indefinitely …eventually we will need to develop a financing system that is sustainable in the long run. Such a system will inherently alter the process by which new innovation moves into medical practice" (Ref. 6, p. 37). Precision health technologies, given their often steep prices, presage exacerbation of this challenge of ballooning health system expenditures.

The health sector also underscores the moral challenges presented by innovation and shortage. One of the cruelest manifestations of shortage is the allocation of life-saving technologies only to those who can afford them — and providing economic incentive for innovation focusing on diseases that afflict the rich exclusively, or more than, the poor.[7] The starting point in Kornai and Eggleston[8] is the ethical challenge of promoting individual sovereignty and choice, on the one hand, while assuring social solidarity — i.e., helping the suffering, the troubled and the disadvantaged–on the other. These two ethical principles have their counterparts in the phenomena of innovation and shortage (or access): can a health system sustain both choice (i.e., allowing the wealthy to purchase health improvements, not just flat-screen TVs) *and* solidarity to provide access to those same health improvements for those less fortunate, or at least for what is considered "basic" healthcare? Angus Deaton[2,7] emphasizes a similar point: innovations, first in population health and later in medical care, raised inequality but also brought progress with "trickle down" access for the poor. Certainly a child born today in the poorest country on earth still has a higher potential to live a long healthy life than the richest individuals born over a century ago. This is true because science, population health, and economic development, even if uneven, have expanded the possibilities for all; social policies determine how soon and how completely those same possibilities for healthy longevity are made available to those less fortunate.

The mechanism underlying the "island of shortage" in the health sector bears many similarities to the classic shortage economy symptoms that Kornai has so eloquently and thoroughly dissected.

> Most of the economic environment operates as a surplus economy, with all its usual side effects, but, in the sea of surplus, an island that bears the marks of a shortage economy can be seen. The doctor's office is crowded and you may have to wait for hours. The waiting lists for surgery or diagnostic procedure may be months long (Table 7.1). Patients' freedom is severely restricted in choosing a doctor or a hospital. In fact there are health-care systems that deny patients such freedom entirely, so that they have to accept the assigned doctor or health institution. The concept of forced substitution can also apply in medical care, where patients may not obtain the medicine, treatment, or physician they would choose and have to take what they are allocated (Ref. 1, p. 125).

Such forced substitution may become ever more acute as some patients enjoy access to expensive new personalized medical therapies, while others must make do with older standards of care that eventually will not even qualify as "basic."

But the shortage that drives the health care spending conundrum differs from the generalized shortage under a centrally planned economy. Its effects are similar, but its causes are distinct. Socialist shortage arises without, and indeed stifles, innovation; health sector shortage arises *because of* innovation.

Innovation and shortage are causally and inextricably intertwined in the health sector, representing a Yin and Yang cycle: shortage spurs innovation, innovation breeds shortage, which in turn already provides the seeds of new innovations. Whether ultimately this is a virtuous or vicious cycle depends on the wisdom of policy choices.

To be more specific, the high price of new therapies and devices exacerbates shortage, but can also serve to prod the same or other innovators to search for lower cost ways of producing and delivering the innovations, as well as pressure for policy innovations to support access. Egalitarian distribution blunts incentives for innovation by reducing the rewards innovators can charge high willingness-to-pay consumers; however, the commitment to egalitarian distribution in the health sector also encourages innovation, because it (1) reassures innovating firms that their products will have a ready market (eventually), rather than be permanently relegated to the niche market of only the richest population; and (2) spurs cost-reducing innovations in new technologies.

Thus, the shortage manifest within health systems, particularly in high-income capitalist economies but throughout the world to greater or lesser extent, is itself a product of surplus. It is only because the economy — in the same country, or elsewhere on the globe — is constantly producing breakthrough technologies for health and medical care that the health policymakers in a given country continually face a dilemma regarding financing access to those innovations. This stream of new health technologies prompts governments to create agencies to evaluate their costs and benefits, a topic we turn to next.

Evaluating innovations and mitigating shortage: Health technology assessment agencies

Given the Yin and Yang of innovation and shortage in the health sector, formal institutions for weighing benefits and costs of new health interventions and medical technologies have emerged in both low- and high-income countries over the past two decades. Starting with some initial studies and policy decisions in the US, other countries have pioneered in the use of cost-effectiveness for health system decision making. Most prominent is the UK, with its NICE (now National Institute for Health and Care Excellence) established in 1999. Australia instituted health economic assessment for pharmaceuticals even earlier. Canadian law articulates "resources stewardship" as a principle guiding the health system, and government agencies and/or formal requirements for health technology assessment with cost-effectiveness analyses have been established in Sweden (2002), Germany (2004), France (2005), Netherlands (2005), Poland (2005 Agency for Polish Technology Assessment), South Korea (2006), and in multiple countries in other regions.[10,11] In Japan, the government decided in 2014 to launch a pilot program for health technology assessment, and by 2017 several pharmaceuticals had been reviewed in this cost-effectiveness appraisal process. Moreover, prominent organizations in global health, both public and private, have embraced the need for systematic presentation of costs as one input to decision making for health.[11]

The trend has not been uniformly towards greater acceptance of such institutions. In the US, the Office of Technology Assessment, established in 1972, was abolished by Congress in 1995, just when health technology assessment agencies were being launched in other countries. In fact, the 2010 Affordable Care Act in the US proscribes use of cost-effectiveness thresholds.

Interestingly, the explicit consideration of costs has been less controversial and more widespread for preventive services and health and occupational safety regulation, compared to curative medical therapies. This tendency might not appear surprising in light of the differences people perceive in allocating resources for saving "statistical lives" versus identified lives (individuals with names facing life-or-death choices).

Among medical technologies, the most common and earliest applications have been for pharmaceuticals, as pioneered by Australia a quarter century ago. When a society refuses to use explicit cost-effectiveness analyses, such as in the US for most beneficiaries of public or private insurance coverage, then the function of allocating access falls to price: what co-payments insured patients must pay, or the full prices set for therapies not covered by insurance at all. Pharmaceutical pricing illustrates this dilemma of promoting access (favoring a low, marginal cost price) versus incentives for innovation (favoring a higher, above-average-cost price). Without past innovation, there can be no current access; and pricing for current innovators will determine what access is possible in the future. No pricing policy can achieve both the dynamic efficiency of covering joint sunk costs of research and development and some return on investment, while simultaneously promoting broad access (static efficiency) with prices not much higher than user-specific marginal costs of production. Some policies, such as patent protection, generic promotion, and compulsory licensing, try to balance the imperatives, mitigating the innovation-inspired shortage.

Examples from Precision and Personalized Medicine (PPM)

Precision medicine has a range of definitions, but in general refers to tailoring interventions or therapies to an individual's characteristics as assessed by biomarkers, often genetic testing, that predict the individual's response to a specific treatment. More generally, precision and personalized medicine (PPM) connotes combination of a therapy with a companion diagnostic test to identify the individuals who would respond to the therapy.[12]

Personalized medicine dominates in the newest anti-cancer treatments. It is no coincidence that some of the more recent countries or regions to adopt cost-effectiveness criteria in decision-making have focused on assessment of expensive therapies for cancer, such as Japan's pilot program. New precision medicine technologies such as genomic diagnostic tests and targeted therapies often promise great clinical benefits — substantial gains in survival or even "cures." However, they almost always are extremely expensive.

One of the earliest and most well-known examples of PPM is Trastuzumab (Herceptin) for breast cancer. This breakthrough treatment for human epidermal growth factor receptor type 2 (HER2)-positive breast cancer has transformed prognosis for this disease. It uses approved companion diagnostic tests to identify those patients who will respond, including HER2 immunohistochemistry tests and HER2 gene-amplification tests.

Health systems vary in their adoption of this innovative, life-extending technology and its companion diagnostic tests. Herceptin was approved for medical use in the United States in 1998 and in Europe in 2000.[13] Trastuzumab is now on the World Health Organization's List of Essential Medicines, the most effective and safe medicines needed in a health system.[14] According to some sources the wholesale price in the developing world is between 1,800 and 1,955 USD per 440 mg vial,[15] already well below prices in high-income countries but out of reach for the poorest. Even in Australia, a 2001 cost-effectiveness analysis led to rejection for coverage; the government created a separate "Herceptin Program" to provide access for breast cancer patients (Ref. 11, p. 12).

The innovation of trastuzumab begets shortage; some patients do not have access. However, this example also illustrates how, as Deaton[2] emphasizes, the inequality arising from breakthrough technology often leads to later innovations to extend access. In the case of PPM, the development of biosimilars can help to reduce the price and improve access to this technology. Many countries establish systems to try to mitigate shortage and provide access to those otherwise unable to afford the treatment, such as Australia's separate fund covering Herceptin, or Singapore's inclusion of trastuzumab in its medication assistance program.

Shortage, for example as manifest by lack of access to life-extending immune-oncology therapies, spurs cost-reducing innovations, not only in the technologies themselves (e.g., lower-cost diagnostic tests) but also innovations in the institutions created to monitor safety and access (e.g., regulatory approval and insurance coverage decisions).

Innovating firms can also contribute to solidarity-enhancing innovation by designing patient access arrangements to make it possible for poorer patients to receive PPM therapies despite their high price. Actually, such access programs constitute a form of price discrimination — a seller charging different customers different prices for the same good or service. As such, access programs combine social responsibility with profit maximization. In the most common form of price discrimination, a seller differentiates or separates customers into different groups, setting a different price for each group based on certain characteristics such as their willingness and ability to pay, or price elasticity. More inelastic consumers (e.g., the rich) can be charged a higher price than those in the more elastic sub-market (e.g., the poor), leading to more revenue than uniform pricing. The sub-markets must be kept separate to prevent arbitrage by enterprising consumers and their agents (such as US patients buying online drugs at prices offered in poor countries); the separation can be enforced by time, physical distance, and/or nature of use. Of course a prerequisite for price discrimination is that the seller possesses a monopoly or at least some market power to set prices.

Pharmaceutical firms' patient assistance programs illustrate how price discrimination reduces shortage and enhances access for the poor. The firm can separate the low-income patients eligible for the assistance program from the "average" patient covered by health insurance, charging the latter a price well above marginal cost....

CONCLUSION

The incorporation of personalized medicine into clinical practice represents a long-term trend that interacts with demographic changes to challenge current and future generations. Longer lives and higher proportions of older people may exacerbate shortage, despite the tremendous product and service innovations that Kornai has emphasized spring from the dynamism of capitalism. The irony seems profound[8]: Is the good or service that we value most — health and longevity — ironically the one where we cannot enjoy the surplus economy of capitalism? Ultimately the answer to this question depends on whether we can innovate with cost-reducing products and strategies as much as with cost-increasing ones, and are resiliently persistent in our quest to balance choice with solidarity.

Cautious optimism could be warranted regarding the power of innovation to produce both "miracle drugs" and the new approaches to financing and payment that will spread their benefits more widely. Public and private sector stakeholders have to work together to enhance access while avoiding conflicts of interest.... In the health sector, dangers arise from over-emphasizing the Yin of innovation over the Yang of access, and vice versa. If we over-constrain innovation, we die needlessly early and forfeit quality of life that innovations might have enabled. If we do not distribute access to innovations equitably, we diminish our humanity, suffer backlashes from populism and distrust of science and expertise, and risk social instability, even violent conflict.[*] Wisely navigating these dangerous shoals will determine whether or not our children and grandchildren have the opportunity to live healthy lives to 100 years old and beyond.

REFERENCES

1. Kornai, János (2013). *Dynamism, Rivalry, and the Surplus Economy: Two Essays on the Nature of Capitalism.* Oxford University Press: Oxford, UK.
2. Deaton, Angus. (2013). *The Great Escape: Health, Wealth, and the Origins of Inequality.* Princeton, NJ: Princeton University Press.
3. Babiarz, Kimberly Singer, Eggleston, Karen, Miller, Grant and Zhang, Qiong. (2015). "An exploration of China's Mortality Decline under Mao: A provincial analysis, 1950–1980." *Population Studies* **69**(1): 39–56.
4. Nobelprize.org. (12 October 2017). "Youyou Tu — Facts." Nobel Media AB 2014. Web. http://www.nobelprize.org/nobel_prizes/medicine/laureates/2015/tu-facts.html.
5. Arrow, K. J. (1963). "Uncertainty and the Welfare Economics of Medical Care." *American Economic Review* **53**(5): 941–973.
6. Chernew, Michael E. and Newhouse, Joseph P. (2012). "Health Care Spending Growth." *Handbook of Health Economics* **2**: 1–43.
7. Deaton, Angus. (2003). "Health, Inequality, and Economic Development." *Journal of Economic Literature* **41**(1): 113–158.
8. Eggleston, Karen. (2016). "Innovation, Shortage, and the Economics of Health Care Systems." In *Constraints and Driving Forces in Economic Systems: Studies in Honour of János Kornai*, eds. Balazs Hamori and Miklos Rosta. Cambridge, UK, Cambridge Scholars Publishing, pp. 15–29.

---

[*] Clearly, those who insist all health care is a "human right" do not usually mean they condone bankrupting taxpayers and eviscerating efforts to address the social determinants of health to provide access to any medical technology that provides a few extra hours of comfort; and those who want to reward innovation while insisting the poor and sick can wait for "trickle down benefits" cannot deny the ethical challenges of consigning to early death those patients with rapidly progressing life-threatening conditions like cancer.

9. Kornai, János and Eggleston, Karen. (2001). *Welfare, Choice and Solidarity in Transition: Reforming the Health Sector in Eastern Europe.* Cambridge, UK, Cambridge University Press, Vietnamese edition (2002), Polish edition (2003), Chinese edition (2003), Hungarian edition (2004).
10. Gulácsi, L., Orlewska, E. and Péntek, M. (2012). "Health Economics and Health Technology Assessment in Central and Eastern Europe: A Dose of Reality." *The European Journal of Health Economics* **13**(5): 525–531. https://link.springer.com/article/10.1007%2Fs10198-012-0411-x.
11. Neumann, Peter J., Ganiats, Theodore G., Russell, Louise B., Sanders, Gillian D. and Siegel, Joanna E. eds. (2017). *Cost Effectiveness in Health and Medicine.* Oxford University Press: Oxford, UK.
12. Berndt, Ernst R. and Trusheim, Mark R. (September 2017). "The Information Pharms Race and Competitive Dynamics of Precision Medicine." Paper Presented at the National Bureau of Economic Research Conference on Economic Dimensions of Personalized and Precision Medicine, Santa Monica, CA.
13. European Medicines Agency. "Herceptin." EMA.europa.eu. Last Updated April 19, 2017. http://www.ema.europa.eu/ema/index.jsp?curl=pages/medicines/human/medicines/000278/human_med_000818.jsp&murl=menus/medicines/medicines.jsp&mid=WC0b01ac058001d125 (Accessed September 5, 2017).
14. World Health Organization. (April 2015). "19th WHO Model List of Essential Medicines." https://www.who.int/groups/expert-committee-on-selection-and-use-of-essential-medicines/essential-medicines-lists.
15. Management Sciences for Health. (January, 2014). "Trastuzumab." MSHpriceguide.org. Accessed September 5, 2017. http://mshpriceguide.org/en/single-drug-information/?DMFId=1471&searchYear=2014.

We Can't Have Everything: The Role of Payment for Volume and Choice of Providers in Fueling Health Care Expenditures

VICTOR R. FUCHS

Stanford University, Stanford CA, USA

President Biden's administration faces a plethora of major domestic and international problems; priorities must be established. The most urgent task is to end the COVID-19 pandemic and provide relief for those who have been most adversely affected by it. Subsequently, another high priority should be ending the increase in health care expenditures' share of the total economy, which has grown to almost 18 percent, from 4.6 percent in 1950. Continuation of this trend would create major budget crises for the federal and state governments; result in stagnant wages and higher taxes for millions of middle class households; and hurt the poor in particular by decreasing the money available for government funding of income support, social services, and public transportation.

Over the last 70 years, national health expenditures (NHE) have increased at an average rate of 4 percent per annum; the gross domestic product (GDP) has increased at 2 percent per annum. (Both rates are per capita adjusted for inflation by GDP deflator.) As long as NHE increases more rapidly than GDP, NHE's share of GDP will get larger. At some point, the need for higher taxes and more debt will put the entire U.S. economy at risk.

To control health care expenditures, several health policy reforms are necessary. Important among these, policymakers must confront the fact that the

Originally published in the *Health Affairs* Forefront on April 28, 2021, available at https://www.healthaffairs.org/do/10.1377/forefront.20210427.833824/full/.

interaction between insured patients' free choice of providers and payment for volume (i.e., fee-for-service) can be toxic for efforts to restrain spending. The stimulus to expenditures from this interaction can be seen clearly in community hospitals. Except during the pandemic, U.S. community hospitals have had an average occupancy rate of 65 percent. Most also have high overhead. Many compete for insured patients with the newest technology, more clinical staff per patient, rooms that offer more space and privacy, deluxe meals, and other amenities. This "race to the top" affects expenditures like an elevator that only goes in one direction-up.

In health policy as in life, we can't have everything; we must decide what we are willing to give up. Below, I discuss several reform options, each of which involves sacrificing some aspects of complete consumer freedom to some extent. I also consider the obstacles to major health policy reform in the United States.

WHAT CAN BE DONE?

The role of health insurance

Health insurance increases the demand for care, but eliminating insurance is not a viable option because of its value to patients and providers. Except for routine checkups and childbirth, individual need for care is usually uneven and unpredictable. Most patients do not have enough cash or money market funds to pay for such care in a timely fashion.

Moreover, in any given year, health care bills are concentrated on relatively few patients. In 2017, only 5 percent of patients accounted for more than 50 percent of expenditures. Without insurance, many of those patients would be financially ruined and some physicians and hospitals would not get paid. Deductibles and copays decrease demand for care, but they exacerbate income inequality because they burden lower-income households more than their higher-income counterparts.

Regulating fee for service

Fee-for-service payment doesn't always result in very high expenditures, as demonstrated in France, Germany, Japan, and several smaller countries that pay for physician visits that way. These governments embed their physician payment in extensive cost controls through various combinations of low fixed-fee schedules, expenditure limits, regulation of the number and specialty mix of physicians, and other policies. Such government intrusion into the private practice of medicine would probably not be workable or acceptable in the United States.

Competing capitated plans

A significant alternative to fee-for-service insurance is a system that pays health plans a risk-adjusted capitation fee for each person enrolled in a plan; the fee covers physician care, hospital care, drugs, tests and scans, and other clinical services. Patient choice is limited to providers in the plan, but annual open enrollment provides the opportunity to choose among plans. Within a plan, patients can choose their primary care physician — a good match results in greater patient satisfaction and possibly better outcomes. Choice of surgeon within a plan also has psychological benefits; although several surgeons of equal skill may be available, many patients think that the one they chose is the "best," and this belief may contribute to better outcomes.

This type of plan, which combines insurance with comprehensive care, is spreading, especially in public insurance such as Medicare Advantage and Medicaid. (Traditional Medicare, which covers 60 percent of beneficiaries, allows free choice of providers and pays for volume.) There is resistance to such plans in some areas of the country, and they are more difficult to organize where population density is low.

Obstacles to major reform

Large scale change in the almost one-fifth of the economy represented by the health care sector would inevitably result in "winners" and "losers." Political experts from Machiavelli to the present have concluded that those who expect to lose from a change will oppose it more vigorously than those who think they might gain will support it. Most affluent households prefer the U.S. system to those in other high-income countries because it offers (1) easier access to specialists and subspecialists; (2) more abundant supplies of expensive medical technologies, unconstrained by national cost-benefit standards; and (3) payment for care through employment-based insurance rather than tax-financed public insurance.

Also benefiting from the current system are manufacturers of drugs, devices, and equipment who earn above-normal profits from the system's emphasis on new medical technologies. Many communities resist change because the local hospital is the largest employer. Many specialist physicians resist change because their fees are at least double those of their peers in other high-income countries.

Major reform is also opposed by millions of workers who mistakenly believe that employers bear the cost of so-called "employer-provided" insurance. Most economists believe that workers actually bear the cost in the form of stagnant wages. Trends over the last 25 years strongly support that conclusion. Between 1991–1993 and 2016–2018, health insurance premiums increased 150 percent while the wages of the median worker increased only 28 percent. By contrast, the earnings of the Standard and Poor's 500 companies have increased 200 percent. (All statistics adjusted for inflation by GDP deflator.)

Many beneficiaries of public insurance also misperceive the cost of these programs. They think that their care is a "free gift" from the government. They don't realize that the increasing cost of care adversely affects government funding of social programs that are of great value to them. A one percentage point increase in health care's share of GDP means there is $200 billion less every year for other goods and services that might do more for health of the poor than the increase in health care expenditures.

The U.S. political system with its "checks and balances" is also a barrier to large scale change: There are many "choke points" ranging from a subcommittee vote to table a reform bill to a presidential veto. It may require a political crisis resulting from a world war, a depression, or large-scale civil unrest to overcome the "status quo." Some experts believe that the COVID-19 pandemic will provide the political shock needed for major health care reform. That is uncertain, and control of expenditures should be more prominent in the suggested reforms. Another political obstacle can arise when those favoring reform cannot agree on a compromise regarding improvements in access, cost, and quality of care. Diverse supporters of reform must also agree on a balance between a much larger role for government and changes in incentives and other reforms of the private sector.

LOOKING FORWARD

Despite these obstacles, future increases in health care expenditures' share of GDP will pressure the system to change. Minor adjustments will be suggested, but they will be like treating cancer with pain killers. Government price controls could provide short-term symptomatic relief but would delay treating the systemic problems that are responsible for the high cost of care.

In comparison with health care systems in other high-income countries, U.S. health care is too costly (18 percent of GDP rather than 12 percent), too unequal, and comes with too much uncertainty about insurance eligibility and coverage. Limiting but not eliminating patient choice of provider, and limiting or preferably replacing payment for volume, should both be part of the solution. A system of competing, capitated plans offering comprehensive care is the most promising vehicle for the United States to reform its health care system and control health care spending.

CONCLUSION

Stabilizing Health Care's Share of the GDP

JONATHAN SKINNER, PH.D.
Dartmouth College, Hanover NH, USA
ELI CAHAN, M.S.
New York University, New York NY, USA
VICTOR R. FUCHS, PH.D.
Stanford University, Stanford CA, USA

The increase in U.S. national health care expenditures from 4 percent of the gross domestic product (GDP) in 1950 to nearly 18 percent of the GDP in 2019 is one of the most important economic changes that occurred in the United States during this period. Since the 1980s, policymakers and private health insurers have implemented interventions aimed at "bending the cost curve," including diagnosis related group-based payments to hospitals, managed care, deductibles and copayments, and bundled-payment programs. But the long-term growth of health care expenditures as a share of the GDP has continued (see Figure 1). Since 1960, health care's share of the GDP has risen by an average of 2.2 percentage points per decade, as compared with an average increase of 1.1 percentage points per decade in 15 other high-income countries since the early 1970s (when the Organization for Economic Cooperation and Development [OECD] began tracking these data; see the Supplementary Appendix, available at NEJM.org).

Increases in health care's share of the GDP in the United States haven't been uniform in the short term. In some years, increases have been higher than average (such as during the creation of Medicare and Medicaid in the 1960s), whereas in other years, they have been lower than average (such as during managed care expansion in the 1990s and in the 2010s). The longer-term trend has been remarkably (and statistically) stable, however: the per-decade growth in health care's

Originally published in NEJM.org on February 19, 2022.

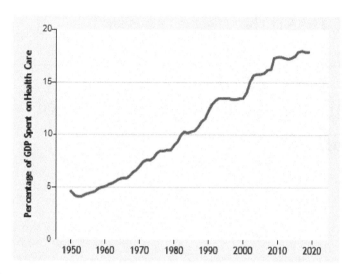

Figure 1

Ratio of National Health Expenditures to GDP, 1950 to 2019.

Source: Data are from the U.S. Social Security Administration 1976 Compendium of National Health Expenditures Data and the Federal Reserve Economic Data database at the Federal Reserve Bank of St. Louis. GDP denotes gross domestic product.

share of the GDP was 1.8 percentage points between 1960 and 1979, then 2.3 percentage points between 1980 and 1999, as well as 2.3 percentage points between 2000 and 2019.

WHY SHOULD THIS RAPID AND PERSISTENT GROWTH BE CONCERNING?

Research has demonstrated that nearly all wage and salary increases between 1999 and 2009 for the median-income American worker were absorbed by increases in health care premiums, out-of-pocket expenses, and taxes to fund Medicare and Medicaid, which has resulted in little left over for discretionary purchases or savings.[1] There is also no evidence that life expectancy has improved more rapidly among Americans than among people in comparable countries, despite higher health care expenditures in the United States.

We believe that a sustainable long-term economic strategy should involve stabilizing the ratio of national health care expenditures to GDP. This goal could be achieved by focusing on the gap between the rate of growth of health care expenditures and the rate of GDP growth. When the gap between these growth rates is greater than zero, health care's share of the GDP rises over time; to stabilize the ratio of health care expenditures to GDP, expenditure growth must be equal to (or less than) GDP growth, which has averaged 3.0 percent per year since 1960 after adjustment for inflation. Focusing on this gap as a target for health policy provides a transparent goal, with results that can be easily measured and monitored. Moreover, if the goal isn't met, it's readily apparent how much change is required to meet it. The potential savings associated with stabilizing the growth of health care expenditures are considerable. If health care's share of the GDP were to be stabilized at 18 percent beginning in 2022, total health care expenditures (in 2021 dollars) between 2022 and 2031 would be $52 trillion, according to Congressional Budget Office projections. In contrast, if health care's share of the GDP continued to grow at the same rate as it has since 1980 (2.3 percentage points per decade), total expenditures would be higher by approximately $3 trillion — money that could instead be spent on addressing social determinants of health by means of investments in education, social services, and improved living standards.

How should the United States approach the goal of restraining the growth of health care expenditures? Various strategies have been proposed for cutting spending, such as limiting out-of-network or "surprise" billing, restricting the delivery of fraudulent postacute care, and expanding preferred pharmacy networks.[2] Although reducing wasteful spending is an important goal, targeting the gap in growth rates requires strategies that can slow the rate of growth of health care expenditures more generally.

A key reason for high rates of growth in this sector is the lack of institutional budgets to constrain spending. Medicare is an entitlement program without legislative limits on expenditures; hospitals respond to rising costs by increasing commercial prices, and increases are passed on to consumers in the form of higher insurance premiums. Medicaid, which is subject to state-level budget constraints, is an exception; perhaps as a consequence, Medicaid has had stable per enrollee inflation-adjusted spending during the past several decades.[3]

In contrast, many OECD countries have fixed budgets for health care organizations that are implicitly tied to tax revenue and general economic growth. Similar approaches could be adopted in the United States. Governments and private insurers, for example, could provide capitated payments to hospitals and physician practices to help them pay their fixed costs of operation, with annual increases tethered to GDP growth. These subsidies would create an environment under which per service prices could be reduced (by means of either competition or regulation), thereby reducing incentives for over-use. Subsidies would also promote financial solvency when visits and admissions fall, as they did during the early stages of the COVID-19 pandemic. Such methods have already demonstrated promise: a global budget has been the hallmark of Maryland's approach to controlling hospital costs.[4] Greater reliance on capitated spending also ensures that providers have incentives to allocate scarce health care resources more effectively. When health care budgets are tied to general economic growth, the result is a stable ratio of health care expenditures to GDP. Slowing the growth of health care expenditures doesn't need to mean restricting research and development.

Most biomedical research and development in the United States focuses on product improvement, with little attention paid to cost reduction; the Food and Drug Administration is forbidden by law from considering cost when evaluating new medical technologies.[5] Other U.S. industries and health care systems in other countries have a more balanced approach, which includes standardized and rigorous use of cost-effectiveness analyses. For example, in England, the National Institute for Health and Care Excellence is required to consider cost in its evaluation of new medical technologies.

The stabilization goal we propose has several caveats. First, health care probably doesn't need to consume as much as 18 percent of the GDP; other high-income countries have effective health care systems that are popular across the political spectrum and consume 12 percent of their GDPs or less. Scaling back health care's share of the GDP would face extraordinary political obstacles, however. Second, year-to-year fluctuations in the GDP's rate of change are greater than would be desirable for health care. One solution would be to link target health care expenditures to average GDP growth over the previous 3 to 5 years. Third, new and expensive innovations may strain health care budgets, but reallocation of health care dollars from less effective to more effective products and services is an essential feature of any sustainable health care system. Fourth, balancing budgets doesn't ensure high-quality health care; further efforts would be necessary to improve clinical quality. Finally, slowing the rate of growth of health care expenditures is likely to remain politically unpopular so long as voters don't connect reduced growth with more reasonable medical bills and insurance premiums.

One might view the COVID-19 pandemic as a challenge to our proposed limits on health care spending; the ratio of health care expenditures to GDP rose to 18.2 percent in 2020, even after subtracting federal COVID-19 supplemental funding. We acknowledge such challenges, associated with temporary increases in health care spending (or with temporary declines in the GDP), but failing to stabilize the long-term ratio of health care expenditures to GDP could result in stagnant wages for most American workers; an increase in bankruptcies among patients, with associated unpaid physician and hospital bills; and budget crises for the federal government and state governments. We believe that stabilizing health care's share of the GDP using transparent, effective, and practical measures should be a national priority.

Disclosure forms provided by the authors are available at NEJM.org.

REFERENCES

1. Auerbach, D. I. and Kellermann, A. L. (2011). "A Decade of Health Care Cost Growth has Wiped Out Real Income Gains for an Average US Family." *Health Affairs (Millwood)* **30**: 1630–1636.
2. Cooper, Z. and Scott Morton, F. (2021). "1 Percent Steps for Health Care Reform: Implications for Health Care Policy and for Researchers." *Health Services Research* **56**: 346–349.

3. Colla, C. and Skinner, J. (2020). "Has the Affordable Care Act Made Health Care More Affordable?" In *The Trillion Dollar Revolution: How the Affordable Care Act Transformed Politics, Law, and Health Care in America*, eds. E. Emanuel and A. Gluck. PublicAffairs: New York, pp. 250–263.

4. Aliu, O., Lee, A. W. P., Efron, J. E., Higgins, R. S. D. and Butler, C. E. (2021). "Offodile AC II Assessment of Costs and Care Quality Associated with Major Surgical Procedures after Implementation of Maryland's Capitated Budget Model." *JAMA Network Open* **4**(9): e2126619.

5. Cahan, E. M., Kocher, B. and Bohn, R. (June 4, 2020). "Why isn't Innovation Helping Reduce Health Care Costs?" *Health Affairs Blog*. https://www.healthaffairs.org/do/10.1377/hblog20200602.168241/full/.

ONLINE APPENDIX

Stabilizing Health Care's Share of the Gross Domestic Product

JONATHAN SKINNER, PH.D.
Dartmouth College, Hanover NH, USA
ELI CAHAN, M.A.
New York University, New York NY, USA
VICTOR R. FUCHS, PH.D.
Stanford University, Stanford CA, USA

DATA

Our measure of NHE adjusts for both population growth and general price inflation. Nominal aggregate U.S. NHE comes from the Centers for Medicare and Medicaid Services (CMS) from 1960 to 2019 (the most recent year available), with data from 1950–1959 derived from the Social Security Administration's 1976 Compendium of National Health Expenditures Data. We adjust for inflation using the GDP Deflator, and population growth, using data from the Federal Reserve Economic Data (FRED) at the Federal Reserve Bank of St. Louis.

Data on Gross Domestic Product (GDP) was also derived from the FRED database, adjusted similarly for inflation using the implicit GDP deflator, and expressed in per-capita terms. In the analysis of changes over time, we use natural logarithms; for example, the 20-year GDP growth rate for 1999–2019 is the difference between the natural log of GDP in 2019 and the natural log of GDP in 1999 (and expressed in percentage terms), adjusted for population growth and inflation.

Average annual rates of change in the ratio of NHE to GDP during 1980–2000 were not significantly different from the corresponding rate of change between 1960–1980 (p-value 0.40) nor for 2000–2019 (p-value 0.56). To test for an arbitrary break in the annual growth rate, we use the Supremum Wald test testing for any break; the p-value was 0.10.

As comparison countries, we used data from the Organisation for Economic Co-Operation and Development (OECD) for European countries and Canada, where the criterion for inclusion was whether there was data on the ratio of NHE to GDP since at least 1972 (a few countries were missing data for 1970 or 1971). The Table presents annual changes in the ratio of NHE/GDP and annual changes in life expectancy; in the text we report annual and decadal changes (e.g., over 10 years) for the change in NHE/GDP.

One may view these overall life expectancy rates as a crude measure of health care quality, as life expectancy likely reflects a variety of other factors not directly related to the health care system. However, other comparisons that attempt to focus more precisely on outcomes related to the quality of health care find that (for example) even those Americans living in the wealthiest counties experience no better health outcomes than the average European high-income country.[1]

THE RELATIONSHIP BETWEEN THE CHANGE IN NHE/GDP AND THE NHE "GAP"

While the paper does not go into much detail on the relationship between the change in NHE/GDP and the NHE gap, there is a close mathematical association that we describe here.

A. *An intuitive approach*: As shown below (in Section B), the percentage point change over time in NHE/GDP is approximately equal to the "gap" (NHE growth minus GDP growth) times the "multiplier" or the ratio NHE/GDP at the beginning of the period. It is easiest to see this using a numerical example:

- NHE as percent of GDP was 18.0 percent in 2016.
- NHE as percent of GDP was 17.6 percent in 2015.

Thus, the change in NHE as a percentage of GDP between 2015 and 2016 was 0.4 percent. Also note that:

- The rate of change in NHE during 2015–2016 was 3 percent.
- The rate of change in GDP during 2015–2016 was 0.9 percent

Multiplying the "gap" of 2.1 percent (3.0 percent–0.9 percent) times the initial (fractional) share of NHE to GDP in 2015, 0.176, yields 0.4 percent, or as noted above, the growth in the percent of GDP spent on health care.

This equation demonstrates that so long as NHE growth exceeds GDP growth, the NHE/GDP share will trend upward; only when NHE growth falls short of GDP growth will the NHE share shrink. Finally, the impact of the multiplier — e.g., the initial level of NHE/GDP — means that even a declining (positive) gap, something we observe in the data, can cause the ratio NHE/GDP to grow at a constant or even increasing rate.

COUNTRY	NHE/GDP 1970	NHE/GDP 2019	ANNUAL % CHANGE NHE/GDP 1970–2019	LIFE EXPECTANCY 1970	LIFE EXPECTANCY 2019	ANNUAL CHANGE LIFE EXPECTANCY 1970–2019	STATISTICAL NOTES
Austria	4.84	10.41	0.11	70.0	82.0	0.24	
Belgium	3.86	10.35	0.13	71.1	82.1	0.22	
Canada***	6.26	10.79	0.09	72.1	82.1	0.20	
Denmark*	7.68	10.03	0.05	73.3	81.5	0.17	
Finland	4.99	9.09	0.08	70.8	82.1	0.23	
France	5.20	11.19	0.12	72.2	82.9	0.22	Break in series
Germany	5.71	11.65	0.12	70.6	81.4	0.22	Break in series
Ireland	4.91	6.84	0.04	71.2	82.8	0.24	
Netherlands**	5.59	9.97	0.09	73.7	82.2	0.18	
Norway	3.99	10.49	0.13	74.4	83.0	0.18	
Portugal	2.26	9.56	0.15	66.7	81.8	0.31	
Spain	3.14	9.00	0.12	72.0	83.9	0.24	
Sweden	5.47	10.88	0.11	74.8	83.2	0.17	
Switzerland	4.90	12.14	0.15	73.1	84.0	0.22	
United Kingdom	3.97	10.25	0.13	71.9	81.3	0.19	
United States	6.25	16.96	0.22 2.2% per decade	70.9	78.9	0.16	1.6 years per decade
OECD Average (excl. US)	4.85	10.18	0.11 1.1% per decade	71.9	82.4	0.22	2.2 years per decade

Expenditures: * From 1971; ** From 1972. Life expectancy: *** from 1971.

Sources: OECD statistics 2020 (NHE), 2021 (Life Expectancy).

B. *A more formal derivation*: Let M_t be national health expenditures (NHE) in year t, and Y_t denote gross domestic product (GDP) also in year t. Taking a first-order Taylor-series approximation, the temporal change in the ratio M_t/Y_t is written:

$$\Delta\left(\frac{M_t}{Y_t}\right) \cong \left[\frac{\Delta M_t}{Y_t} - \frac{M_t \Delta Y_t}{Y_t^2}\right] \tag{A.1}$$

Rearranging to express as proportional (or log) change yields:

$$\Delta\left(\frac{M_t}{Y_t}\right) \cong \left(\frac{M_t}{Y_t}\right)\left[\frac{\Delta M_t}{M_t} - \frac{\Delta Y_t}{Y_t}\right] \tag{A.2}$$

Table: Projections of Real National Healthcare Expenditures (NHE) 2022–2031 under Two Scenarios: A Constant (18%) Ratio of NHE to GDP, and a Growing Ratio (18% to 20.1%) of NHE to GDP.

YEAR (1)	CBO GDP PROJECTIONS (REAL 2021 DOLLARS) (2)	NHE WHEN NHE/ GDP REMAINS CONSTANT AT 18% FRACTION (3)	NHE/GDP FRACTION GROWS BY 2.3 PERCENTAGE POINTS PER DECADE (4)	IMPLIED NHE WITH GROWING FRACTION (5)
2021	$22,974	$4135		
2022	24,120	4435	0.180	$4435
2023	24,490	4602	0.182	4660
2024	24,756	4753	0.185	4874
2025	25,069	4916	0.187	5104
2026	25,427	5092	0.189	5353
2027	25,845	5287	0.192	5625
2028	26,249	5485	0.194	5905
2029	26,651	5686	0.196	6194
2030	27,067	5894	0.198	6497
2031	27,524	6117	0.201	6821
TOTAL NHE	2022–2031	$52,267		$55,468
			DIFFERENCE	$3,202

Note: Numbers are in billions of constant (2021) dollars. NHE denotes National Healthcare Expenditures.

This means that when health expenditure growth is more rapid than GDP growth, the share of GDP devoted to health care will rise by the initial share times the gap in relative growth rates, and conversely.

PROJECTED SAVINGS RESULTING FROM STABILIZING THE GROWTH IN HEALTH EXPENDITURES RELATIVE TO GDP

The table shows projected GDP from 2021 to 2031 according to Congressional Budget Office estimates published in July 2021.[2] Real calendar GDP is calculated from the CBO statistical supplement (cited above) but normalized to 2021 prices.

We assume that the ratio of NHE to GDP is 18 percent in 2022, and consider health spending under a constant 18 percent rate from 2022–2031 (Column 3), which is just Column 2 (GDP) times .18, compared to a ratio that is growing at the rate of 2.3 percentage points per decade (Column 4), leading to health care spending rising at a more rapid rate (Column 5). Total inflation-adjusted spending with a constant 18 percent share is $52.3 trillion, for the rising share it is $55.5 trillion; the difference is $3.2 trillion.

REFERENCES

1. Emanuel, E. J., Gudbranson, E., Van Parys, J., Gørtz, M., Helgeland, J. and Skinner, J. (2021). "Comparing Health Outcomes of Privileged US Citizens with those of Average Residents of other Developed Countries." *JAMA Internal Medicine* **181**(3): 339–344.
2. Congressional Budget Office (2021). "An Update to the Budget and Economic Outlook: 2021 to 2031, July." https://www.cbo.gov/system/files/2021-07/57218-Outlook.pdf.

Part 3
Summary of Years 2012–2021

SUMMARY OF YEARS 2012–2021

THE AFFORDABLE CARE ACT (ACA) AND THE UNINSURED

The ACA ("Obamacare") offered financial incentives to the states to expand their Medicaid programs, provided subsidies for low-income individuals to purchase private insurance through state-administered insurance exchanges, prohibited insurance companies from denying coverage for previous existing conditions, mandated insurance for some firms, and had other less consequential provisions. It was signed into law in 2010 but was not "fully" implemented until 2014. "Fully" is in quotes because by 2016 only 33 states plus DC, accounting for 64 percent of the U.S. population, had exercised the ACA option to expand Medicaid.

Despite only partial implementation, between 2013 and 2016, there was a huge decrease in the percent of the population without health insurance. Prior to 2014, the uninsured percentage was relatively stable in the range of 14 percent to 15 percent. It began to decrease sharply in 2014 and continued to decrease until 2016, when it stabilized in the 8 percent to 9 percent range (see Figure ACA1). This decrease between 2013 and 2016 of about 40 percent (6 percentage points in absolute terms) is attributed to the ACA by most experts.[2,3,11,12,14,15,20,21,31]

Table ACA1 shows that major decreases in the uninsured were experienced between 2013 and 2016 by all ethnic groups. Those groups that had a relatively high percent without insurance in 2013 experienced larger absolute decreases; those groups that had a relatively low percent without insurance in 2013 experienced larger relative decreases. By 2019, over half the uninsured were minorities. Approximately 10 million were Hispanic, 4 million were Black, and 1 million were Asian. Because Medicare provides insurance for nearly all individuals age 65 and over, almost all of the reduction in uninsured between 2013 and 2016 was experienced by the under 65 age group (see Table ACA2).

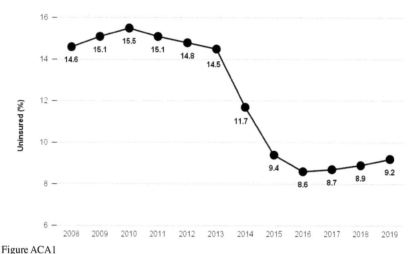

Figure ACA1

Percent of population with no health insurance coverage, 2008–2019

Source: U.S. Census Bureau, 2008 to 2019 American Community Surveys (ACS).

Table ACA1. Percent of ethnic group with no health insurance in 2013 and 2016.

| | PERCENT WITH NO INSURANCE | | CHANGE FROM 2013 TO 2016 | |
| | | | ABSOLUTE | RELATIVE |
ETHNIC GROUP	2013	2016	(PERCENTAGE POINT)	(PERCENT)
American Indian & Alaskan Native	26.9	19.2	−7.7	−28.6
Hispanic	26.4	18.0	−8.4	−31.8
Native Hawaiian and other Pacific Islander	17.9	9.9	−8.0	−44.7
Black	17.1	9.7	−7.4	−43.3
Asian	14.6	7.8	−6.8	−46.6
White, not Hispanic	10.2	5.7	−4.5	−44.2
United States	14.4	8.6	−5.8	−40.3

Source: U.S. Census Bureau, 2008–2019 American Community Surveys (ACS). Uninsured by ethnic group reported from "Table HIC9_ACS. Population Without Health Insurance Coverage by Race and Hispanic Origin: 2008–2019," which is based on the race-alone or single-race reporting option, i.e., those who reported Asian and no other race.

HEALTH CARE EXPENDITURES

Health care expenditure (HCE) is the largest category in the economy, absorbing almost 18 percent of the Gross Domestic Product (GDP). It is three times as much as the country spends on education, and almost five times the expenditures on national defense. In 2019, the last year before the COVID-19

Table ACA2. Number of uninsured by age in 2013 and 2016.

NUMBER UNINSURED (MILLIONS)	2013	2016	CHANGE (IN MILLIONS) 2013 TO 2016
All ages	45.2	27.3	−17.9
Under 65	44.7	26.9	−17.8
65 and older	0.5	0.4	−0.1

Note: Number uninsured from Health Insurance Historical Tables — HIC ACS (2008–2019) for the civilian non-institutionalized population, available at Census.gov. Number of uninsured 65 and older calculated from total population (HIC4) less persons age 65 (HIC6), i.e., "Table HIC–4_ACS, Health Insurance Status and Type of Coverage by State All Persons: 2008–2019," and "Table HIC–6_ACS, Health Insurance Coverage Status and/type of Coverage by State-Persons Under 65:2008–2019."

Source: U.S. Census Bureau, 2008 to 2019 American Community Surveys (ACS).[33]

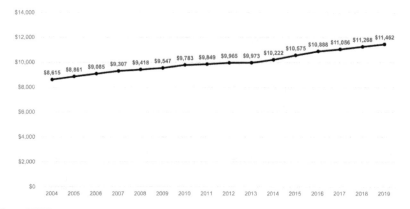

Figure HCE1

Annual per capita health care expenditures (HCE), 2004–2019, in 2019 dollars

Source: National Health Expenditure Accounts NHE2020, Centers for Medicare & Medicaid Services, Office of the Actuary, National Health Statistics Group; and GDP deflator.

pandemic, per capita HCE was $11,462; the national total was $3.8 trillion dollars. Figure HCE1 shows annual per capita HCE in 2019 dollars from 2004 to 2019.[16,19] The change from 2004 to 2011 was 1.9 percent per annum; from 2012 to 2019, it was 2.0 percent per annum.

HCE as a percent of GDP is a useful statistic when comparing changes over time.[32] Figure HCE2 shows changes from 2004 to 2019. The rate of change from 2004 to 2011 was 1.5 percent per annum; between 2012 and 2019, the rate of change was 0.4 percent per annum.

Health care expenditure as a share of GDP in the U.S. has been consistently larger than in other high-income countries for many decades. Table HCE1 compares the U.S. with the ten OECD countries that have the largest HCE/GDP ratios (other than the U.S.). The U.S. level is higher than in every one of the ten other countries and was 1.6 times as high as the average of the ten in 2019.

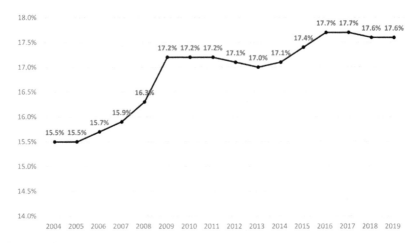

Figure HCE2

Health care expenditures as a share of Gross Domestic Product, 2004–2019

Source: National Health Expenditure Accounts NHE2020, Centers for Medicare & Medicaid Services, Office of the Actuary, National Health Statistics Group; U.S. Department of Commerce, Bureau of Economic Analysis; and U.S. Bureau of the Census.

Table HCE1. Health care expenditures (HCE) as a share of Gross Domestic Product (GDP) in the United States and ten other OECD countries,[a] *2012–2019.*

| | | | CHANGE BETWEEN 2012 AND 2019 | |
| | | | ABSOLUTE | RELATIVE |
COUNTRY	2012	2019	(PERCENTAGE POINTS)	(PERCENT PER ANNUM)
Austria	10.2	10.4	+0.20	+0.28%
Belgium	10.5	10.7	+0.20	+0.27%
Canada	10.5	10.8	+0.34	+0.45%
Denmark	10.2	10.0	−0.29	−0.40%
France	11.3	11.1	−0.19	−0.24%
Germany	10.9	11.7	+0.84	+1.07%
Japan	10.8	11.0	+0.25	+0.32%
Netherlands	10.5	10.2	−0.37	−0.52%
Sweden	10.7	10.9	+0.19	+0.25%
Switzerland	10.2	11.3	+1.04	+1.38%
Average of 10 OECD countries	**10.6**	**10.8**	**+0.22**	**+0.30%**
United States	**17.1**	**17.6**	**+0.50**	**+0.41%**

Note: [a]The ten countries with the highest HCE/GDP ratio after the US.

Source: OECD Health Statistics 2021 and US National Health Expenditure Accounts, Centers for Medicare and Medicaid Services, Office of the Actuary, National Health Statistics Group (which includes investment as well as personal health care expenditures).

The reasons for higher health care expenditures in the U.S. are well known. First and foremost are the large administrative expenses required to run U.S. health care. To call US health care administration a "system" would be an exaggeration. Over one thousand health insurance companies are hired by millions of employers to design, negotiate, and administer distinct health plan contracts with equally numerous hospitals and private practice physicians. Billing and collecting for arbitrarily priced services is a nightmare for most health care providers. No precise figures exist for administrative expenses, but a reasonable estimate is about 25 percent of total health care expenditures — almost one trillion dollars per year.

Second, U.S. prices for brand-name prescription drugs, devices such as hip and knee replacements, and medical equipment are often double what they are in the ten OECD countries. These are apples-to-apples comparisons because the products are identical. It is a classic case of price discrimination. Health product manufacturers rely on the inability of U.S. buyers to acquire the products from other countries at a lower price.

Third, the fees of U.S. physician specialists are often double or triple those of their peers in the ten OECD countries. The comparison is not strictly apples-to-apples because the U.S. physicians usually have more expenses. But the career-long fee differential far outweighs the expense differential on net revenue and results in higher expenditures in the U.S.

A fourth reason for higher HCE/GDP in the U.S. is intercountry differences in the product mix of health care. U.S. medical care puts more emphasis on high technology embodied in expensive diagnostic and therapeutic interventions. Other countries give more emphasis to "high touch" services including more physician visits per capita and more inpatient hospital days per capita. The product mix also varies because the quantity and quality of amenities in the U.S. often exceed those of other countries: U.S. hospital rooms are often more spacious and provide more privacy, meals are more likely to be deluxe, and facilities often feature more consumer technologies.

The fifth reason is that the U.S. system for evaluating new medical technology is biased toward higher expenditures. The Food and Drug Administration is forbidden from considering the cost of a new technology when deciding whether to accept or reject it. The U.K.'s national center for evaluation of medical technology — the National Center for Health and Care Excellence (NICE) — is *required* to consider cost in the evaluation process.

These five reasons why U.S. HCE/GDP is the highest in the world provide a good introduction to explaining why it is politically so difficult to make major changes. Numerous individuals, companies, and organizations expect to be adversely affected financially by major changes in the existing system. In addition, there are many individuals who mistakenly believe that because they have "employer-provided" or "government-provided" insurance, their medical care is free to them. They do not realize that the financial burden of medical care falls on individuals as *workers, consumers, taxpayers*, and members of *households* (particularly low-income households).

By allocating the exceptionally large percentage of human, manufactured, and natural resources to health care, Americans do not realize they are missing out on other potentially more valuable goods and services. For example, if, in the long run, U.S. health care used the same percentage of Gross Domestic Product as the average of the 10 (other) highest spending countries, the U.S. could double spending on education, or build and pay for an additional 3 million dwelling units per year. (The pre-pandemic rate of new units was about 1.3 million per year in 2018–2019.)

HEALTH OUTCOMES

Health is multi-dimensional. There are physical illnesses, mental illnesses, and possible interactions between the physical and the mental. Health problems can be manifest in pain, functional loss, and disability. Measures of health are based on self-reports of patients, diagnoses by physicians, reports by institutions, and administrative records. They are often partly subjective, and can be influenced by changes in laws, insurance coverage, or administrative decisions. The most objective measure of health is mortality, which is important in itself, and is also an indicator of morbidity because most deaths are preceded by illness.

Life expectancy at birth is a useful summary measure of age-specific mortality. It answers the following question: "What would be the average age at death of a cohort born in year X if it experienced the age-specific mortality rates of year X?" Changes in life expectancy at birth (often called "period life expectancy") are used to infer changes in population health; differences in life expectancy between countries or between sub-groups within a country have similar application. Note that when survival is improving over time, the actual lifespan of a given birth cohort ("cohort life expectancy") will be longer than period life expectancy at birth; how much longer depends on future mortality rates.

U.S. life expectancy at birth increased from 65.7 years in 1950 to 76.8 by 2000, an absolute rate of change of approximately +0.2 years per year. The top series in Figure HO1 shows this trend continued after 2000 to about 2010, but then life expectancy at birth abruptly leveled off. In 2019, it was the same as in 2012. The first section of this summary of the years 2012–2021 shows that during 2012–2019 the percent of the population with health insurance increased. The second section shows an increase in real per capita health care expenditures. Historically, health insurance and health care expenditures have been credited with increasing life expectancy, but apparently other factors were at work during 2012–2019.

In high-income countries, more than 8 out of 10 deaths occur after age 65. There is, therefore, considerable interest in life expectancy at age 65, the lower series of Figure HO1. This statistic answers the following question: "For individuals age 65 in year Y, what would be their average additional years of life if they experienced the age-specific mortality rates of year Y?" We see that life expectancy at age 65 rose rapidly until about 2010; after that, it continued to increase but at a much slower rate. The fact that life expectancy at birth was not increasing at a time when life expectancy at age 65 was increasing (albeit slowly) implies that death rates of those under age 65 in 2012–2019 must have been getting worse.

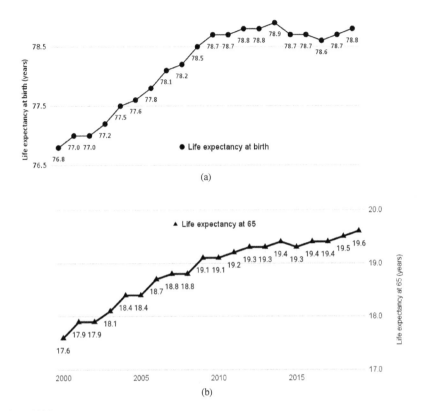

Figure HO1
(a) Life expectancy at birth and (b) at age 65, 2000–2019

Source: National Center for Health Statistics, National Vital Statistics System, mortality; *Health, United States 2019*, Table 4; National Vital Statistics Reports, Vol. 70, No. 8, July 26, 2021, p.75.

Angus Deaton and Anne Case have analyzed this in considerable detail and have concluded that worsening health was particularly true for adults without college degrees. They also emphasize higher age-specific death rates from drug over-doses, alcohol, and suicide, causes that they label "deaths of despair".[5]

Rising mortality for the population under age 65 will be manifest in an increase in the percent of a cohort that does not survive until age 65 and/or a decrease in the average age of death of those who do not survive until 65. Both these series for 2004–2019 are plotted in Figure HO2. The average age of death of those who do not survive until 65 shows small increases or decreases from year to year, but no significant longer-term trends. It was 49.0 years in 2004 and 49.0 in 2018. The percent not surviving until 65 tells a different story. It decreased rapidly from 2004 to 2010, when it abruptly stopped decreasing. It was relatively constant until 2014, and it increased after that. To obtain more understanding of what was hap-pening to mortality under age 65 and its role in life expectancy at birth requires the age distribution of that population for each year and the age-specific mortality

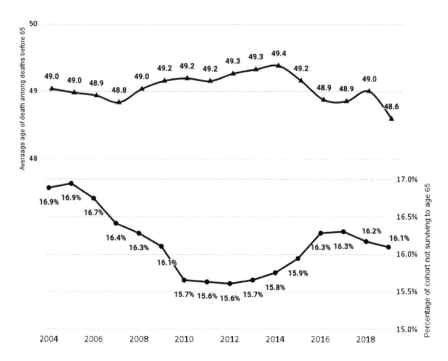

Figure HO2
Percentage who do not survive to age 65 and their average age of death, 2004–2019

Source: National Center for Health Statistics, National Vital Statistics System. Lifetables available at https://www.cdc.gov/nchs/products/life_tables.htm [downloaded February 23 and July 17, 2022]

Table HO1. *Life expectancy at birth and at age 65, by ethnic group, 2006–2019.*

	2006	2011	2012	2019	ABSOLUTE CHANGE PER YEAR 2006–2011	ABSOLUTE CHANGE PER YEAR 2012–2019
Life expectancy at birth						
White non-Hispanic	78.2	78.7	78.9	78.8	+0.10	−0.01
Black non-Hispanic	73.1	75.0	75.1	74.9	+0.38	−0.03
Hispanic	80.3	81.8	81.9	81.8	+0.30	−0.01
Life expectancy at age 65						
White non-Hispanic	18.7	19.1	19.2	19.5	+0.08	+0.04
Black non-Hispanic	17.1	17.9	18.0	18.2	+0.16	+0.03
Hispanic	20.2	21.2	21.4	21.6	+0.20	+0.03

Source: National Center for Health Statistics, National Vital Statistics System, mortality; Health, United States 2019, Table 4. Life expectancy at birth, age 65, and age 75, by sex, race, and Hispanic origin: United States, selected years 1900–2018; National Vital Statistics Reports, Vol. 70, No. 8, July 26, 2021, p. 75, Table I–21. Life expectancy at birth, by race and Hispanic origin and sex: United States, 1940, 1950, 1960, 1970, 1980, 1990, and 2000–2019.

rates for each year. Such detailed data analysis is beyond the scope of this summary of the years 2012–2021 (see National Academies of Sciences, Engineering, and Medicine 2021[24]).

Some additional perspective on life expectancy at birth and at age 65 can be gained through comparing the experience of different ethnic groups within the United States and by comparing the U.S. with other OECD countries. Table HO1 shows that each of the largest ethnic groups (White non-Hispanic, Black non-Hispanic, and Hispanic) had the same experience in 2012–2019. They had no increase in life expectancy at birth and much slower increase in life expectancy at age 65. A comparison of the U.S. experience with the same 10 OECD countries studied in the Health Care Expenditures section shows that in 2012–2019 their life expectancy at birth and at age 65 continued to increase at substantial rates (see Figure HO3 and Table HO2).[10]

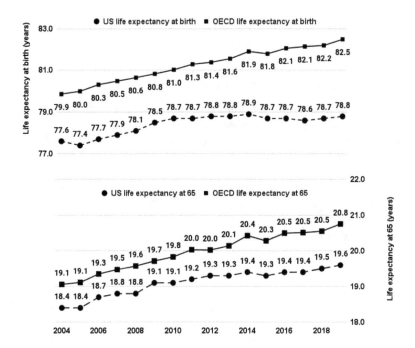

Figure HO3

Life expectancy at birth and at age 65 in the United States and 10 OECD countries, 2004–2019

Note: The OECD averages of life expectancy at birth and at 65 are simple averages for the ten other OECD countries with the highest health spending: Austria, Belgium, Canada, Denmark, France, Germany, Japan, the Netherlands, Sweden, and Switzerland.

Source: National Center for Health Statistics, National Vital Statistics System, mortality; for the other ten OECD countries, Human Mortality Database. Max Planck Institute for Demographic Research (Germany), University of California, Berkeley (USA), and French Institute for Demographic Studies (France). Available at www.mortality.org.

Table HO2. Life expectancy at birth in 10 OECD countries and the United States, 2012–2019.

COUNTRY[a]	2012	2019	ABSOLUTE CHANGE PER YEAR, 2012–2019
Austria	80.8	81.9	+0.15
Belgium	80.3	81.8	+0.23
Canada	81.7	82.4	+0.09
Denmark	80.1	81.4	+0.19
France	81.8	82.8	+0.14
Germany	80.5	81.2	+0.10
Japan	83.2	84.5	+0.18
Netherlands	81.1	82.1	+0.14
Sweden	81.7	83.1	+0.19
Switzerland	82.6	83.8	+0.17
Average of 10 OECD countries	**81.4**	**82.5**	**+0.16**
United States	**78.8**	**78.8**	**0.00**

Note: [a]Alphabetical order.

Source: National Center for Health Statistics[25] National Vital Statistics System, mortality; Human Mortality Database (HMD)[17] for the other ten OECD countries.

The principal conclusions of this Health Outcomes section are as follows:

1. In the first decade of the 21st century, life expectancy at birth and at age 65 in the U.S. increased at rates consistent with historical trends.
2. Rather abruptly, at about 2010–2012, life expectancy at birth stopped increasing and the rate of increase at age 65 slowed to less than one-half its previous rate.
3. The same changes in life expectancy at birth and at age 65 were experienced by the three largest ethnic groups: White non-Hispanic, Black non-Hispanic, and Hispanic.
4. These changes were **not** experienced by peer countries in the OECD.

THE COVID-19 PANDEMIC

In late 2019 in Wuhan, China, a virus not previously seen in humans appeared. (Subsequently, the disease caused by this virus became known as COVID-19.) On January 19, 2020, in Sonomish County, Washington, a patient was diagnosed with an infection attributed to this virus. On January 31, 2020, in Santa Clara County, California, a patient was hospitalized for COVID-19 and died on February 6. On March 11, 2020, the World Health Organization declared COVID-19 a global pandemic. In the U.S., the pandemic disrupted most households and brought death to many. It forced millions of business firms, schools, and non-profit organizations to close their doors or radically readjust their operations. It overwhelmed health care systems in many areas of the country to the breaking point, and resulted in an unprecedented increase in the national death rate. This section describes and briefly discusses these traumatic changes by comparing data for 2018 and 2019 with 2020. The calendar years do not correspond exactly with the absence or presence of the COVID-19 pandemic, but they are close. We treat the changes from 2018 and 2019 to 2020 as useful indicators of changes from pre-pandemic to pandemic conditions.

In 2020, the first year of the COVID-19 pandemic, life expectancy fell drastically. Life expectancy at birth was 1.75 years below the average of 2018 and 2019 and the percent per annum rate of decrease was 1.50 (Table CP1). The rate of decrease of life expectancy at age 65 was 3.68 percent per annum. These were extraordinarily rapid rates of change for life expectancy which usually changes gradually. Over the last 60 years, the average rate of increase in life expectancy at birth was approximately 0.2 percent per annum.

Table CP1 shows that the pandemic was particularly traumatic for Black and Hispanic life expectancy. Compared with the average of 2018 and 2019, life expectancy at birth fell 1.2 years for Whites, but 3.1 years for Blacks and 3.0 years for Hispanics. Likely explanations for the ethnic differences include greater transmission of the virus for Blacks and Hispanics because of denser populations in their households and neighborhoods, a higher percentage of Blacks and Hispanics

Table CP1. Life expectancy at birth and at age 65 in the U.S. and three major ethnic groups, 2018, 2019, 2020.

| | | | | CHANGE FROM AVERAGE OF 2018 AND 2019 TO 2020 | |
| | | | | ABSOLUTE (YEARS PER ANNUM) | RELATIVE (PERCENT PER ANNUM) |
	2018	2019	2020		
Life expectancy at birth					
Total population	78.7	78.8	77.0	−1.17	−1.50%
White non-Hispanic	78.7	78.8	77.6	−0.77	−0.98%
Black non-Hispanic	74.9	74.9	71.8	−2.07	−2.82%
Hispanic	81.8	81.8	78.8	−2.00	−2.49%
Life expectancy at age 65					
Total population	19.5	19.6	18.5	−0.70	−3.68%
White non-Hispanic	19.4	19.5	18.8	−0.43	−2.27%
Black non-Hispanic	18.0	18.2	16.6	−1.00	−5.77%
Hispanic	21.4	21.6	19.8	−1.13	−5.49%

Sources: National Center for Health Statistics, National Vital Statistics System, mortality; National Vital Statistics Reports, Vol. 70, No. 8, July 26, 2021, p. 75, Table I–21; Table. Provisional expectation of life, by age, Hispanic origin, race for the non-Hispanic population, and sex: United States, 2020. In Arias E, Tejada-Vera B, Ahmad F, Kochanek KD. Provisional life expectancy estimates for 2020. Vital Statistics Rapid Release; no 15. Hyattsville, MD: National Center for Health Statistics. July 2021. https://dx.doi.org/10.15620/cdc:107201; Murphy SL, Kochanek KD, Xu JQ, Arias E. Mortality in the United States, 2020. NCHS Data Brief, no. 427. Hyattsville, MD: National Center for Health Statistics. 2021. https://dx.doi.org/10.15620/cdc:112079.

Table CP2. Life expectancy at birth in ten high-income OECD countries compared with the U.S., 2018, 2019, 2020.

	2018	2019	2020	CHANGE FROM AVERAGE OF 2018 AND 2019 TO 2020	
				ABSOLUTE (YEARS PER ANNUM)	RELATIVE (PERCENT PER ANNUM)
Austria	81.8	82.0	81.3	−0.40	−0.49%
Belgium	81.7	82.1	80.9	−0.67	−0.82%
Canada	82.0	82.1	81.7	−0.23	−0.28%
Denmark	81.0	81.5	81.6	+0.23	+0.29%
France	82.8	82.9	82.3	−0.37	−0.44%
Germany	81.0	81.4	81.1	−0.07	−0.08%
Japan	84.3	84.4	84.7	+0.23	+0.28%
Netherlands	81.9	82.2	81.5	−0.37	−0.45%
Sweden	82.6	83.2	82.5	−0.27	−0.32%
Switzerland	83.8	84.0	83.2	−0.47	−0.56%
Average of ten OECD countries	82.3	82.6	82.1	−0.24	−0.29%
United States	78.7	78.8	77.0	−1.17	−1.50%

Sources: Murphy SL, Kochanek KD, Xu JQ, Arias E. Mortality in the United States, 2020. NCHS Data Brief, no 427. Hyattsville, MD: National Center for Health Statistics. 2021. DOI: https://dx.doi.org/10.15620/cdc:112079; OECD Health data.

working in occupations that could not be transformed to remote work, Blacks and Hispanics being less likely to be able to move to residences with less exposure to COVID-19, and worse access to medical care for Blacks and Hispanics, which may have become more of a liability under pandemic conditions.[1]

The pandemic started in China but quickly spread globally. Other high-income countries in the OECD were much more effective than the U.S. in limiting its impact on life expectancy, as shown in Table CP2 and Figure CP1. The 10 OECD countries that we used for comparison with the U.S. in previous sections because of their relatively high ratio of health care expenditures to gross domestic product were used to compare life expectancy. Before the pandemic, the U.S. was frequently criticized for having lower life expectancy than the other high-income countries,[26] but the differential became much larger in 2020. In 2018 and 2019, Americans had 3.6 years less life expectancy than their peers in the average of the 10 OECD countries. After the pandemic struck, that widened to 5.1 years in 2020. We consider possible explanations for the larger effect of the pandemic on the U.S. in the last section of this summary of the years 2012–2021 where we discuss politics, government, and health.

In the U.S. in 2020, there were 536,768 more deaths than in the average of 2018 and 2019. Federal government researchers who analyzed the cause of death designated on state death certificates found COVID-19 was the stated cause in 65 percent of the deaths and other causes in 35 percent (Centers for Disease Control and Prevention,

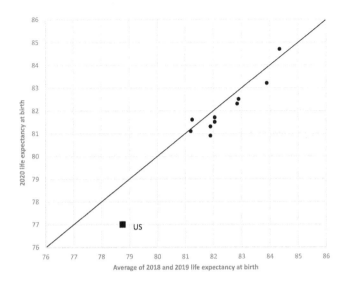

Figure CP1

Life expectancy at birth, US and 10 other OECD countries, 2020 compared to 2018–2019 average

National Center for Health Statistics. National Vital Statistics System, Mortality 2018–2020, on CDC WONDER Online Database, released in 2021). Commentators have noted, however, that the pandemic was probably an indirect cause of many of these other deaths as well.[6,13,22,27,28] Some individuals with life-threatening illness did not receive timely and appropriate care because medical personnel and institutions were overwhelmed with caring for COVID-19 patients. Other sick individuals may not have sought care in time because they feared contact with medical care would increase their chance of being infected by COVID-19. The number of individuals with some other cause on their death certificates who did not seek or get needed care because of the pandemic is not known. Several researchers have different estimates of the total number of what they label "excess" deaths attributable to COVID-19 and the substantial ethnic, socioeconomic, and geographic differences in those deaths (Figure CP2).[22,27,28]

Table CP3 provides additional information about deaths in 2020 by comparing changes from 2018 and 2019 for selected causes of death. By focusing on rates of change of causes of death, we can see that 2020 was very different from the pre-pandemic years. The number of deaths from all causes surged at a rate of 11.5 percent per annum. By historical standards, this is a huge change in rates. The average rate of increase of the number of deaths over the last 50 years has been 1.2 percent per annum.

For many decades, heart disease and malignant neoplasms (cancer) have been the leading causes of death. In 2018 and 2019, their combined share of all causes

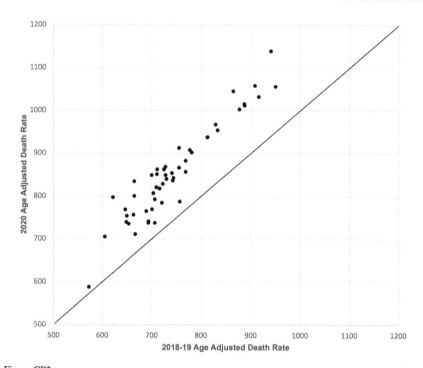

Figure CP2

Age-adjusted death rate, US States, 2020 compared to 2018–2019 average

Note: For related research and discussion, see Refs. 7,8,10.

Source: Centers for Disease Control and Prevention, National Center for Health Statistics. Underlying Cause of Death 1999–2020 on CDC WONDER Online Database, released in 2021. Data are from the Multiple Cause of Death Files, 1999–2020, as compiled from data provided by the 57 vital statistics jurisdictions through the Vital Statistics Cooperative Program. Accessed at http://wonder.cdc.gov/ucd-icd10.html on May 4, 2022.

of death was 44 percent. In 2020, their combined share was 38 percent. That's not because there were fewer deaths from the two causes. The increase for malignant neoplasm was very small but heart disease deaths increased by 4 percent per annum. Their combined absolute increase, however, accounted for only 8 percent of the absolute increase in deaths from all causes.

Deaths from drug overdoses ("deaths of despair" highlighted by Case and Deaton) and from guns present a different picture. Their combined rate of increase from the average of 2018 and 2019 was 15.2 percent per annum. The opioid epidemic had been underway for several years, and there probably would have been an increase in drug overdoses as a cause of death even if there were no pandemic. Whether the pandemic exacerbated the increase in drug overdoses, and if so, by how much, is not known. The increase in gun deaths is not well understood, but a large increase in gun supply probably contributed.

Table CP3. Deaths from select causes, 2018, 2019, 2020.

	2018	2019	2020	CHANGE FROM AVERAGE OF 2018 AND 2019 TO 2020 (ABSOLUTE PER ANNUM)	(PERCENT PER ANNUM)
Deaths					
All causes	2,839,205	2,854,838	3,383,729	357,805	11.5
Heart diseases	655,381	659,041	696,962	26,501	3.92
Malignant neoplasms	599,274	599,601	602,350	1,942	0.32
(Combined)	1,254,655	1,258,642	1,299,312	28,442	2.23
Drug overdoses	71,147	74,511	96,096	15,511	18.5
Guns[a]	39,740	39,707	45,222	3,666	8.64
(Combined)	110,887	114,218	141,318	19,177	15.2
COVID-19	0	0	350,831	233,887	NA
Other causes	1,473,663	1,481,978	1,592,268	76,298	4.97

Note: [a]Firearm-related deaths, e.g., suicides and homicides involving guns, from vital statistics as summarized by Johns Hopkins Center for Gun Violence Solutions (2022).

Note that the age-adjusted death rates for heart disease and cancer were declining pre-2020, a trend that reversed significantly for heart disease in 2020. For cancer, the age-adjusted death rate in 2020 was slightly lower than in the preceding two years.

Sources: Centers for Disease Control and Prevention, National Center for Health Statistics. National Vital Statistics System, Mortality 2018–2020 on CDC WONDER Online Database, released in 2021; Gun deaths from CDC as summarized by Johns Hopkins Center for Gun Violence Solutions.[18]

The biggest change in 2020 was a new cause of death: COVID-19. Of the increase in deaths from all causes of 536,702, deaths with COVID-19 as the cause totaled 350,381. There were no known COVID-19 deaths in the U.S. in 2018 or 2019; it is, therefore, impossible to calculate a percent per annum rate of change to 2020. It is also arbitrary to calculate an absolute rate of change per annum. We have assumed a rate (233,887) which is two-thirds of the total COVID-19 deaths, the same as the absolute rate per annum for all-cause mortality. The conclusion that COVID-19 was the major reason for increased deaths in 2020 is independent of this assumption. Indeed, the full impact of the pandemic on the increase in deaths in 2020 was probably much greater than 65 percent, but how much greater is not known. The "other causes" category had a 5 percent increase which included causes that increased in importance and a few that decreased. The combined high rate of change probably included causes that were adversely affected by the pandemic.

To further explore the background of the pandemic, Table CP4 focuses on American households in 2018, 2019, and 2020. Pre-pandemic, most American households were in a relatively good economic condition. The share of households

Table CP4. Household circumstances in 2020 compared with 2018 and 2019.

| | | | | CHANGE FROM AVERAGE OF 2018 AND 2019 TO 2020 | |
	2018	2019	2020	(ABSOLUTE PER ANNUM)	(PERCENT PER ANNUM)
Percentage of households in poverty	9.00	7.80	8.70	0.20	2.34
White households in poverty (%)	5.80	5.00	5.80	0.27	4.76
Black households in poverty (%)	17.7	16.3	16.8	–0.13	–0.79
Hispanic households in poverty (%)	15.5	13.9	14.8	0.07	0.45
Median household income (2020 dollars)	65,127	69,560	67,521	118	0.18
Earnings of median full-time worker (2020 dollars)	52,472	52,650	56,287	2,484	4.57
Personal disposable income (billions of constant dollars)	14,429	14,755	15,673	720	4.76
Personal consumption expenditures (billions of constant dollars)	12,845	13,126	12,630	–237	–1.85
Remote work (%)	4.80	4.80	49.9	30.1	156
In-person schooling (%)	100	100	43.1	–38.0	–56.2
Pandemic-related transfers from the government to households (billions of dollars)	0	0	3,094	NA	NA
Population (millions)	329	331	332	1.43	0.43
Number of households (millions)	83.5	83.7	83.9	0.20	0.24
Number of homeless (to Jan. 2020 only)	552,830	567,715	580,466	13,462	2.36
Consumer Price Index	1.50	1.80	1.50	–0.10	–6.35

Notes: Note that the data series for remote work represents the percentage of full paid working days from home, using the Barrero *et al.* (2021) estimates. The pre-pandemic figure of 4.8 percent is based on their analysis of the 2017–2018 American Time Use Survey; the 2020 figure represents the average of the monthly work-from-home estimates for all months of data collected during 2020 (May through December). School learning mode data from Burbio, fall 2020 average, with hybrid instruction (2–3 days per week in-person) weighted 50 percent and traditional (5-days in person) weighted at 100 percent; data available and further definitions provided at https://cai.burbio.com/school-opening-tracker/. The pandemic-related transfers from the government to households include Economic impact payments; Lost wages supplemental payments; Provider Relief Fund and Paycheck Protection Program loans to nonprofit institutions serving households; Pandemic Unemployment Compensation Payments; Pandemic Unemployment Assistance; Pandemic Emergency Unemployment Compensation, and Extended Unemployment Benefits.

Sources: U.S. Bureau of Economic Analysis; Shrider, Emily A., Melissa Kollar, Frances Chen, and Jessica Semega, U.S. Census Bureau, Current Population Reports, P60–273, Income and Poverty in the United States: 2020, U.S. Government Publishing Office, Washington, DC, September 2021; Federal Reserve Economic Data: FRED. Federal Reserve Bank of St. Louis; The Economic Report of the President 2022, appendix tables; for remote work, Barrero, Jose Maria, Nicholas Bloom, and Steven J. Davis, 2021. "Why working from home will stick," National Bureau of Economic Research Working Paper 28731. School learning mode data from Burbio, fall 2020 average, https://cai.burbio.com/school-opening-tracker/; U.S. Department of Housing and Urban Development, Annual Homeless Assessment Report to Congress, Point-In-Time count and Housing Inventory Count conducted in January 2020.

in poverty in 2018 was 9 percent, and it fell further to 7.8 percent in 2019. Median household income was $65,127 in 2018 and $69,560 in 2019. The pandemic in 2020 was disruptive to households in many ways; but the gross measures of economic well-being did not change much. The percent of households in poverty increased slightly, primarily for white households, not Black or Hispanic. Median household income in 2020 was slightly above the average of 2018 and 2019.

Table CP5. Household behavior in 2020 compared with 2018 and 2019.

	2018	2019	2020	CHANGE FROM AVERAGE OF 2018 AND 2019 TO 2020	
				(ABSOLUTE PER ANNUM)	(PERCENT PER ANNUM)
Marriages	2,132,853	2,015,603	1,676,911	−264,878	−14.2
Divorces	782,038	746,971	630,505	−89,333	−12.8
Movie theaters (revenues, millions of dollars)	74,000	74,972	65,854	−5,755	−8.21
Hotels and motels (revenues, millions of dollars)	193,160	200,890	116,127	−53,932	−35.2
Full-service restaurants (billions of dollars)	318	334	254	−47.9	−16.6
Limited-service restaurants (billions of dollars)	321	341	330	−0.90	−0.27
Vehicle miles traveled (millions of miles)	269,995	271,770	241,907	−19,317	−7.54
Airline use	84,365,157	88,021,676	33,134,274	−35,372,762	−63.7

Notes: Note that airline use is measured as "Revenue Passenger Miles for U.S. Air Carrier Domestic and International, Scheduled Passenger Flights, in thousands)" and movie theater revenues is "Total Revenue for Motion Picture and Video Production and Distribution, All Establishments, Employer Firms, Millions of Dollars, Annual."

Source: Federal Reserve Economic Data: FRED. Federal Reserve Bank of St. Louis.

The difference in what happened to disposable personal income and personal consumption expenditures in 2020 is interesting. The former increased but the latter decreased. The buildup of savings set the stage for demand outpacing supply in 2021. Probably the most important change for households was the closing of schools and the increase of work from home.

Table CP5 describes some changes in household behavior in 2020 probably related to the pandemic. There was substantial decline in marriages (minus 14 percent per annum), but also a decline in divorce (minus 13 percent). The absolute decline in marriages was three times as great as the absolute decline in divorce. In response to pandemic-induced lockdowns, masking and social distancing restrictions, and fear of a COVID-19 infection, there were reductions in revenues of movie theaters, hotels, motels, and restaurants. Interestingly, the effect on restaurant revenues was felt only in "full service" ones (server takes an order and brings meal to table). Limited-service restaurants (e.g., McDonalds) that do a large "take out" business had little change in revenues. The effect on airline use was huge; there was also some decrease in vehicle use, but much less.

Table CP6 presents a few important macroeconomic indicators to suggest how the overall economy fared in 2020 relative to 2018 and 2019. Most indicators were down, but not by much. Per capita GDP in constant dollars fell by 2 percent per annum. The index of industrial production fell by 5 percent per annum. The employment/population ratio declined 2.5 percentage points; the unemployment

*Table CP6. Select macroeconomic indicators in 2020 compared with
2018 and 2019.*

	2018	2019	2020	CHANGE FROM AVERAGE OF 2018 AND 2019 TO 2020	
				(ABSOLUTE PER ANNUM)	(PERCENT PER ANNUM)
GDP per capita (Chained 2012 dollars)	56,591	57,585	55,415	−1,115	−1.98
Index of industrial production	103.2	102.3	95.0	−5.17	−5.23
Civilian employment/population ratio	60.4	60.8	56.8	−2.53	−4.32
Labor force participation (%)	62.9	63.1	61.8	−0.80	−1.28
Unemployment rate	3.9	3.7	8.1	2.87	50.5
S&P 500 stock price index	2746	2913	3218	259	8.57
Profits of S&P 500 companies	39.0%	48.3%	47.6%	2.63%	5.78
GDP Price Deflator (2019=100)	98.2	100	101.2	1.40	1.40

Sources: Federal Reserve Economic Data (FRED), Federal Reserve Bank of St. Louis; the Economic Report of the President 2022, Appendix tables; for profits of S&P500 companies, CSI market data on gross margin (csimarket.com).

rate increased by 2.9 percentage points. Company profits and stock prices fared better. The S&P 500 price index was up 8.6 percent The relation between the pandemic and these changes is unclear. The years 2018 and 2019 came after many years of uninterrupted economic expansion — from 2010 to 2018 and 2019, the unemployment rate fell from 9.6 to 3.9 and 3.7 percent; the S&P 500 price index rose from 1258 to 2746 and 2913. Some readjustment might have occurred in 2020 in the absence of the pandemic. For the economy as a whole, 2020 was a year of conflicting trends. Many industries experienced declines in revenues, but the federal government provided substantial financial stimulus to households and firms.[4]

HEALTH AND POLITICS

This section begins by extending the discussion of the COVID-19 pandemic to focus on the difference between the individual states and the ten individual OECD countries. Table HP1 provides a representative measure of those differences in cumulative COVID-19 deaths per 100,000 population through May 31, 2022. It shows a very large gap between the U.S. states and these ten OECD countries. The median state had almost twice as large a COVID-19 death rate as the median country. Moreover, every state except three (Hawaii, Vermont, and Utah) had a higher death rate than the median country.

This US–OECD difference was not peculiar to the pandemic. An analogous comparison between the individual states and the ten OECD countries for life expectancy at birth in 2018–2019 (Table HP2) reveals a similar large differential. The median life expectancy in the ten OECD countries in 2018–2019 was 82.1 years compared with only 78.5 years in the U.S. Only one state (Hawaii) had a life expectancy greater than the lowest of the ten OECD countries.

Table HP1. Cumulative COVID-19 Deaths per 100,000 (through May 31, 2022) in the United States and 10 High-Income OECD countries.

	MOST	MEDIAN	LEAST	MOST/LEAST
50 U.S. States	419	308	102	4.1
	Mississippi	Kansas	Hawaii	
10 OECD Countries	273	162	24.3	11.2
	Belgium	(Germany 166, Switzerland 158)	Japan	
U.S./OECD	1.53	1.90	4.20	0.37

Source: Johns Hopkins University CSSE COVID-19 Data, downloaded June 2022 from Our World in Data.

Table HP2. Pre-pandemic[a] life expectancy at birth (years) in the United States and 10 high-income OECD countries.

	LOWEST	MEDIAN	HIGHEST	HIGHEST MINUS LOWEST
50 U.S. States	74.5	78.5	81.0	6.5
	West Virginia	Maine, Maryland, Texas	Hawaii	
10 OECD Countries	80.9	82.1	84.4	3.5
	Germany	(Netherlands 81.9, Canada 82.2)	Japan	
OECD minus U.S.	6.4	3.6	3.4	–3.0

Note: [a] Average of 2018 and 2019.

Sources: Centers for Disease Control and Prevention, National Center for Health Statistics. National Vital Statistics System, Mortality 2018–2020 on CDC WONDER Online Database, released in 2021; and Human Mortality Database.

Next, we focus on differences in health outcomes across the individual states in 2012, the average of 2018–2019, and the cumulative COVID-19 death rate in the 2020s. The correlation over time between different state-level measures of health outcomes is quite high. Between cumulative COVID-19 death rates and life expectancy in 2012, the coefficient is –0.60. And between cumulative COVID-19 death rates and average life expectancy in 2018 and 2019, it is also –0.60. The coefficient of correlation between life expectancy in 2012 and the average of 2018 and 2019 is +0.98.

Because of the high interest in political party preferences and polarization, we also focus on the Republican presidential candidate *vote share* in the 2012, 2016, and 2020 elections. Correlation over time in Republican vote share across the states was even higher than for health outcomes: between 2012 and 2016, +0.96; between 2012 and 2020, +0.95; and between 2016 and 2020, +0.99.

More importantly, the correlation between the Republican presidential candidate vote share and health outcomes is highly significant (see Table HP3). If the data are arrayed and ranked, the coefficient of rank correlation between the Republican candidate vote share and health outcomes is high, regardless of time period (Table HP4).

Table HP3. Coefficient of correlation between health outcomes and Republican presidential candidate vote share across states in three time periods.

	REPUBLICAN PRESIDENTIAL CANDIDATE VOTE SHARES		
	2012	2016	2020
Life expectancy 2012	−0.4807	−0.5018	−0.5267
Life expectancy average 2018 & 2019	−0.4799	−0.5187	−0.5373
Cumulative COVID-19 deaths (to May 31, 2022)	+0.3896	+0.4332	+0.4600

Note: Life expectancy refers to life expectancy at birth. The 2012 state lifetables come from the United States Mortality Data Base (USMDB, available at https://usa.mortality.org/) and the 2018 and 2019 state lifetables are from the US National Center for Health Statistics. The Republican presidential candidate vote share is the share of votes relative to the total votes of the two major political party candidates, from the UC Santa Barbara American Presidency Project, https://www.presidency.ucsb.edu/.

Table HP4. Coefficient of rank correlation between health outcomes and Republican presidential candidate vote share across states in three time periods.

	REPUBLICAN PRESIDENTIAL CANDIDATE VOTE SHARES (RANKS)		
HEALTH OUTCOMES (RANKS)	2012	2016	2020
Life expectancy 2012 (lowest to highest)	+0.5602	+0.5777	+0.5934
Life expectancy average 2018 & 2019 (lowest to highest)	+0.5459	+0.5815	+0.5874
Cumulative COVID-19 deaths (to May 31, 2022, highest to lowest)	+0.3698	+0.4217	+0.4419

Three additional observations are important to keep in mind when interpreting the strong negative correlation (−0.65) between life expectancy and the Republican presidential candidate vote share. First, the relation was as strong in 2012 as in 2016 and 2020 when Donald Trump was the Republican candidate. Second, states differ substantially in average level of education. The percentage of age 25+ with a bachelor's degree or higher is positively correlated with life expectancy (+0.80) and negatively correlated with Republican vote share (−0.83). Third, states differ substantially in attitudes and legislation about many social issues, such as abortion. Polarization is partially due to strong differences across the country in these social and cultural issues that some people feel are essentially religious or fundamental to their identity. A Pew Research Center state by state survey about making abortion illegal (except in rare cases) was negatively correlated with life expectancy (−0.74) and positively correlated with Republican vote share (0.81); see Figure HP1. To attempt to infer causal relationships from such a complex set

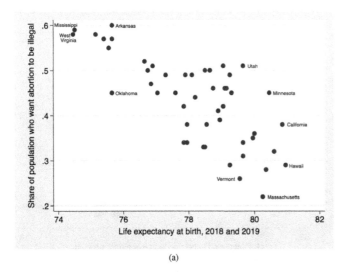

(a)

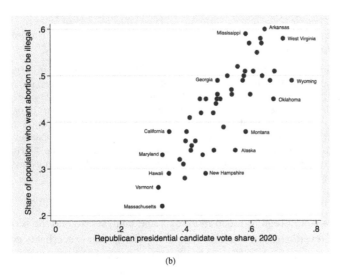

(b)

Figure HP1

Life expectancy, Republican presidential candidate vote share, educational attainment, and abortion attitudes across states.

(a) Life expectancy (average of 2018 and 2019) and share of state population saying abortion should be illegal (except in rare cases); (b) Republican presidential candidate vote share in 2020 and share of state population saying abortion should be illegal (except in rare cases); (*Continued*)

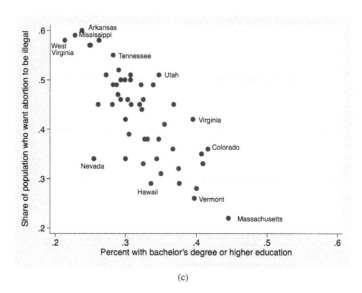

(c)

Figure HP1 (*Continued*)
(c) Share of state population with bachelor's degree or higher education (in 2020) and share of state population saying abortion should be illegal (except in rare cases)

Note: Life expectancy refers to life expectancy at birth. The 2012 state lifetables come from the United States Mortality Data Base (USMDB, available at https://usa.mortality.org/) and the 2018 and 2019 state lifetables are from the US National Center for Health Statistics. The Republican presidential candidate vote share is the share of votes relative to the total votes of the two major political party candidates, from the UC Santa Barbara American Presidency Project, https://www.presidency.ucsb.edu/. Data for share of state population who say abortion should be illegal in all/most cases from Pew 2014 U.S. Religious Landscape Study, conducted June 4–Sept. 30, 2014, which surveyed 35,000 U.S. adults across 50 states (no data for D.C.). For further discussion of these associations, see Refs. 9,23,27,29,30

of variables would require much more data and analysis beyond the scope of this overview. Nevertheless, it is clear that party polarization exacerbates conflicts of interest (mentioned when discussing health care expenditures) and makes any large-scale changes in health policy politically difficult.

REFERENCES
1. Alsan, Marcella, Chandra, Amitabh and Simon, Kosali. (2021). "The Great Unequalizer: Initial Health Effects of COVID-19 in the United States." *Journal of Economic Perspectives* **35**(3): 25–46.
2. Baumgartner, Jesse, Collins, Sara, Radley, David and Hayes, Susan (2020). "How the Affordable Care Act (ACA) has Narrowed Racial and Ethnic Disparities in Insurance Coverage and Access to Health Care, 2013–2018." *Health Services Research* **55**: 56–57.
3. Busch, Susan H., Golberstein, Ezra and Meara, Ellen (August 2014). "ACA dependent coverage provision reduced high out-of-pocket health care spending for young adults." *Health Affairs* (Project Hope) **33**(8): 1361–1366. https://doi.org/10.1377/hlthaff.2014.0155.

4. CARES Act (Coronavirus Aid, Relief, and Economic Security Act), Pub. L. 116–136 (2020).

5. Case, Anne and Deaton, Angus (2020). *Deaths of Despair and the Future of Capitalism*. Princeton University Press: Princeton, NJ, USA.

6. CDC. (2021). "Excess Deaths Associated with COVID-19." https://www.cdc.gov/nchs/nvss/vsrr/covid19/excess_deaths.htm.

7. Couillard, Benjamin K., Foote, Christopher L., Gandhi, Kavish, Meara, Ellen and Skinner, Jonathan (2021). "Rising Geographic Disparities in US Mortality." *Journal of Economic Perspectives* **35**(4): 123–146.

8. Currie, Janet and Schwandt, Hannes (2016) "Mortality Inequality: The Good News from a County-level Approach." *Journal of Economic Perspectives* **30**(2): 29–52.

9. DellaVigna, Stefano and Kim, Woojin (June 2022). "Policy Diffusion and Polarization across U.S. States." NBER Working Paper No. 30142.

10. Deryugina, Tatyana and Molitor, David (2021). "The Causal Effects of Place on Health and Longevity." *Journal of Economic Perspectives* **35**(4): 147–170.

11. Dranove, David, Garthwaite, Craig and Ody, Christopher (August 1, 2016). "Uncompensated Care Decreased at Hospitals in Medicaid Expansion States but not at Hospitals in Nonexpansion States." *Health Affairs* **35**(8): 1471–1479. https://doi.org/10.1377/hlthaff.2015.1344.

12. Duggan, Mark, Goda, Gopi Shah and Li, Gina (June 1, 2021). "The Effects of the Affordable Care Act on the Near Elderly: Evidence for Health Insurance Coverage and Labor Market Outcomes." *Tax Policy and the Economy* **35**: 179–223. https://doi.org/10.1086/713496.

13. *The Economist*. "The Pandemic's True Death Toll: Our Daily Estimate of Excess Deaths around the World." https://www.economist.com/graphic-detail/coronavirus-excess-deathsestimates.

14. Glied, Sherry A., Collins, Sara R. and Lin, Saunders (2020). "Did the ACA Lower Americans' Financial Barriers to Health Care? A Review of Evidence to Determine Whether the Affordable Care Act was Effective in Lowering Cost Barriers to Health Insurance Coverage and Health Care." *Health Affairs* **39**(3): 379–386.

15. Goldin, Jacob, Lurie, Ithai Z. and McCubbin, Janet (2021). "Health Insurance and Mortality: Experimental Evidence from Taxpayer Outreach." *The Quarterly Journal of Economics* **136**(1): 1–49.

16. Hartman, Micah, Martin, Anne B., Washington, Benjamin, Catlin, Aaron and National Health Expenditure Accounts Team (2022). "National Health Care Spending in 2020: Growth Driven by Federal Spending in Response to the COVID-19 Pandemic: National Health Expenditures Study Examines US Health Care Spending in 2020." *Health Affairs* **41**(1): 13–25.

17. Human Mortality Database (HMD). *Max Planck Institute for Demographic Research (Germany)*. University of California: Berkeley (USA), and French Institute for Demographic Studies (France). www.mortality.org.

18. Johns Hopkins Center for Gun Violence Solutions. (2022). "A Year in Review: 2020 Gun Deaths in the US." https://publichealth.jhu.edu/gun-violence-solutions.

19. Martin, Anne B., Hartman, Micah, Lassman, David, Catlin, Aaron and National Health Expenditure Accounts Team. (2021). "National health care spending in 2019: Steady growth for the fourth consecutive year: Study examines national health care spending for 2019." *Health Affairs* **40**(1): 14–24.

20. Miller, Sarah and Wherry, Laura R. (2019). "Four Years Later: Insurance Coverage and Access to Care Continue to Diverge between ACA Medicaid Expansion and Non-expansion States." In *AEA Papers and Proceedings*, Vol. 109, pp. 327–333.

21. Miller, Sarah, Johnson, Norman and Wherry, Laura R. (2021). "Medicaid and Mortality: New Evidence from Linked Survey and Administrative Data." *The Quarterly Journal of Economics* **136**(3): 1783–1829.

22. Miller, Sarah, Wherry, Laura R. and Mazumder, Bhashkar (August 2021). "Estimated Mortality Increases durthe COVID-19 Pandemic by Socioeconomic Status, Race, and Ethnicity." *Health Affairs* **40**(8): 1252–1260. https://doi.org/10.1377/hlthaff.2021.00414.

23. Mulligan, Casey B. and Arnott, Robert D. (June 2022). "Non-covid Excess Deaths, 2020–2021: Collateral Damage of Policy Choices?" NBER Working Paper No. 30104.

24. National Academies of Sciences, Engineering, and Medicine (2021). *High and Rising Mortality Rates among Working-Age Adults*. The National Academies Press: Washington, DC.

25. National Center for Health Statistics. (May 8, 2022). "Provisional COVID-19 Death Counts by Week Ending Date and State." https://data.cdc.gov/d/r8kw-7aab.

26. National Research Council (2013). *U.S. Health in International Perspective: Shorter Lives, Poorer Health*. The National Academies Press: Washington, DC. https://doi.org/10.17226/13497.

27. Polyakova, Maria, Udalova, Victoria, Kocks, Geoffrey, Genadek, Katie, Finlay, Keith and Finkelstein, Amy N. (February 2021). "Racial Disparities in Excess All-cause Mortality during the Early COVID-19 Pandemic Varied Substantially across States." *Health Affairs* **40**(2): 307–316. https://doi.org/10.1377/hlthaff.2020.02142.

28. Ruhm, Christopher J. (2021). "Excess Deaths in the United States during the First Year of COVID-19." NBER Working Paper No. 29503.

29. Schwandt, Hannes, Currie, Janet, Bär, Marlies, Banks, James, Bertoli, Paola, Bütikofer, Aline, Cattan, Sarah *et al.* (2021). "Inequality in mortality between Black and White Americans by age, place, and cause and in comparison to Europe, 1990–2018." *Proceedings of the National Academy of Sciences* **118**(40): e2104684118.

30. Sehgal, Neil Jay, Yue, Dahai, Pope, Elle, Wang, Ren Hao and Roby, Dylan H. (2022). "The Association between COVID-19 Mortality and the County-level Partisan Divide in the United States: Study Examines the Association between COVID-19 Mortality and County-level Political Party Affiliation." *Health Affairs* **41**(6): 853–863.

31. Soni, Aparna, Wherry, Laura R. and Simon, Kosali I. (2020). "How have ACA Insurance Expansions Affected Health Outcomes? Findings from the Literature: A Literature Review of the AffordCare Act's Effects on Health Outcomes for Non-elderly Adults." *Health Affairs* **39**(3): 371–378.

32. Skinner, Jonathan, Cahan, Eli and Fuchs, Victor R. (2022). "Stabilizing Health Care's Share of the GDP." *The New England Journal of Medicine* **386**(8): 709–711.

33. U.S. Census Bureau, 2008 to 2019 American Community Surveys (ACS). https://www.census.gov/programs-surveys/acs/data.html.

A LOOK TO THE FUTURE

We conclude the third edition of *Who Shall Live?* with deep concern about the future of U.S. health care. If, almost 50 years after the first edition, "high cost," "unequal access," and "disappointing health outcomes" continue to be the system's major problems, what can be expected in the years ahead? No plan for a more efficient, effective, and equitable health care system is currently under discussion. Yet, we know that these problems can be dealt with. Compared with the U.S., other high-income democracies spend one-third less for health care, their populations enjoy three more years of life expectancy, and their health care systems have broad political support.

The current difference in the political situation in the U.S. is particularly problematic. In other countries, health policy is a responsibility that does not depend on which party controls the government. In the U.S., when the Republican Party won control of the federal government in 2016, their principal health policy goal was to repeal Obama's Affordable Care Act. As long as health policy is a political symbol embedded in a polarizing power struggle, significant reform of health care is probably impossible. We can only hope that Alexis de Tocqueville will prove correct when he wrote that American democracy "moves from the impossible to the inevitable without ever stopping at the probable."

Acknowledgments

We are grateful to many institutions, organizations, and individuals who have helped us with this book. These include the Freeman Spogli Institute for International Studies, the National Bureau of Economic Research, and the Stanford Institute for Economic Policy Research. We are also grateful to the organizations and agencies who supplied the data, including the Centers for Disease Control and Prevention National Center for Health Statistics and WONDER Online Database, the U.S. Census Bureau, the Human Mortality Database, the OECD Health Data, and other data sources noted in the text and tables.

We are grateful to the following individuals for their comments, suggestions, and other kinds of assistance: Sandra Berrios, M.D., Mark Cullen, M.D., Ezekiel Emanuel, M.D., Fred Fuchs, Paula Fuchs, Dana Goldman, Yulin Jiang, Rachel Sungyoun Kim, Nancy Fuchs Kreimer, Diego S. Lee, Yoojung Lee, Jimmy Low, Joseph P. Newhouse, Rossannah Reeves, Gregory L. Rosston, Anne Marie Ryschon, Leonard Schaeffer, John B. Shoven, TR Soundararajan, Mele Teu, Richard J. Zeckhauser, Yubing Zhai, Bradley Zlotnick, M.D.

Appendix Table. Data on State Health Outcomes, Republican Presidential Candidate Share of Two Candidates' Votes, Abortion Attitudes, and Educational Attainment

STATE	2012	HEALTH OUTCOMES LIFE EXPECTANCY PRE- PANDEMIC[a]	CUMULATIVE COVID-19 DEATHS[b]	REPUBLICAN CANDIDATE VOTE SHARE 2012	2016	2020	% ABORTION SHOULD BE ILLEGAL IN MOST CASES	EDUCATION (% WITH NO BACHELOR)
Alabama	75.4	75.2	401	0.61	0.64	0.63	0.58	0.738
Alaska	78.2	77.9	170	0.55	0.58	0.55	0.34	0.700
Arizona	79.3	78.8	416	0.54	0.52	0.50	0.46	0.697
Arkansas	75.8	75.7	381	0.61	0.64	0.64	0.60	0.762
California	80.8	80.9	231	0.37	0.34	0.35	0.38	0.653
Colorado	80.3	80.0	221	0.46	0.47	0.43	0.36	0.584
Connecticut	80.9	80.4	307	0.41	0.43	0.40	0.28	0.600
Delaware	78.6	78.0	304	0.40	0.44	0.40	0.38	0.673
District of Columbia	77.9	77.9	190	0.07	0.04	0.06	NA	0.402
Florida	79.5	79.0	347	0.49	0.51	0.52	0.39	0.695
Georgia	77.8	77.3	344	0.53	0.53	0.50	0.49	0.678
Hawaii	81.5	81.0	102	0.28	0.33	0.35	0.29	0.664
Idaho	79.5	79.3	277	0.65	0.68	0.66	0.49	0.713
Illinois	79.1	78.9	301	0.41	0.41	0.41	0.41	0.645
Indiana	77.5	76.9	352	0.54	0.60	0.58	0.51	0.728
Iowa	79.6	79.1	304	0.46	0.55	0.54	0.46	0.707
Kansas	78.6	78.1	308	0.60	0.61	0.57	0.49	0.661
Kentucky	75.8	75.4	356	0.61	0.66	0.63	0.57	0.750
Louisiana	75.8	75.7	373	0.58	0.60	0.59	0.57	0.751
Maine	79.2	78.5	175	0.41	0.48	0.45	0.33	0.675
Maryland	79.3	78.5	241	0.36	0.36	0.33	0.33	0.591
Massachusetts	80.8	80.3	298	0.38	0.35	0.33	0.22	0.555
Michigan	78.2	77.9	364	0.45	0.50	0.49	0.42	0.700
Minnesota	81.0	80.5	229	0.45	0.49	0.46	0.45	0.632
Mississippi	75.1	74.5	419	0.55	0.59	0.58	0.59	0.772
Missouri	77.6	76.8	338	0.54	0.60	0.58	0.50	0.701
Montana	78.9	78.6	318	0.55	0.61	0.58	0.38	0.669
Nebraska	79.6	79.2	221	0.60	0.64	0.60	0.46	0.675
Nevada	78.1	78.0	353	0.46	0.49	0.49	0.34	0.745

Appendix Table. (*Continued*)

STATE	HEALTH OUTCOMES			REPUBLICAN CANDIDATE VOTE SHARE			% ABORTION SHOULD BE ILLEGAL IN MOST CASES	EDUCATION (% WITH NO BACHELOR)
	LIFE EXPECTANCY		CUMULATIVE COVID-19 DEATHS[b]					
	2012	PRE-PANDEMIC[a]		2012	2016	2020		
New Hampshire	80.4	79.3	186	0.47	0.50	0.46	0.29	0.624
New Jersey	80.2	80.0	379	0.41	0.43	0.42	0.35	0.593
New Mexico	77.9	77.1	371	0.43	0.45	0.44	0.45	0.719
New York	80.5	80.6	351	0.35	0.38	0.38	0.32	0.625
North Carolina	78.0	77.6	235	0.50	0.52	0.51	0.45	0.680
North Dakota	79.6	79.1	305	0.58	0.70	0.67	0.51	0.693
Ohio	77.6	76.9	330	0.48	0.54	0.54	0.47	0.711
Oklahoma	75.9	75.7	364	0.67	0.69	0.67	0.45	0.739
Oregon	79.6	79.7	180	0.42	0.44	0.42	0.34	0.656
Pennsylvania	78.5	78.2	353	0.47	0.50	0.49	0.44	0.677
Rhode Island	80.2	79.7	338	0.35	0.42	0.39	0.31	0.650
South Carolina	77.1	76.7	348	0.55	0.57	0.56	0.52	0.710
South Dakota	79.1	78.7	331	0.58	0.66	0.63	0.50	0.707
Tennessee	76.3	75.6	383	0.60	0.64	0.62	0.55	0.718
Texas	78.6	78.5	305	0.57	0.55	0.53	0.50	0.693
Utah	79.9	79.7	149	0.73	0.62	0.61	0.51	0.653
Vermont	80.2	79.6	106	0.31	0.35	0.32	0.26	0.603
Virginia	79.2	79.1	239	0.47	0.47	0.45	0.42	0.605
Washington	80.2	80.0	170	0.41	0.41	0.40	0.36	0.633
West Virginia	75.3	74.5	388	0.62	0.72	0.70	0.58	0.787
Wisconsin	79.7	79.3	251	0.46	0.50	0.50	0.45	0.692
Wyoming	78.5	77.9	314	0.69	0.76	0.72	0.49	0.718

Notes: [a]Average of 2018 and 2019.

[b]Cumulative to May 31, 2022.

Life expectancy refers to life expectancy at birth. The 2012 state lifetables come from the United States Mortality Data Base (USMDB, available at https://usa.mortality.org/) and the 2018 and 2019 state lifetables are from the US National Center for Health Statistics; hence, they are not directly comparable in levels but are useful for comparing dispersion across states at each point in time. The Republican presidential candidate vote share is the share of votes relative to the total votes of the two major political party candidates. Abortion attitudes data extracted from the Pew 2014 Religious Landscape Study (Summary available at https://www.pewresearch.org/fact-tank/2020/01/21/do-state-laws-on-abortion-reflect-public-opinion/).

Index